temptations

IGNITING THE PLEASURE
AND POWER OF APHRODISIACS

BY ELLEN AND MICHAEL ALBERTSON

The Cooking Couple™

D0066982

A FIRESIDE BOOK
Published by Simon & Schuster
New York London Toronto Sydney Singapore

This publication contains the opinions and ideas of its authors. It is intended to provide helpful and informative material on the subjects addressed in the publication. It is sold with the understanding that the authors and publisher are not engaged in rendering medical, health, or any other kind of personal professional services in the book. The reader should consult his or her medical, health, or other competent professional before adopting any of the suggestions in this book or drawing inferences from it.

The authors and publisher specifically disclaim all responsibility for any liability, loss, or risk, personal or otherwise, which is incurred as a consequence, directly or indirectly, of the use and application of any of the contents of this book.

FIRESIDE
Rockefeller Center
1230 Avenue of the Americas
New York, NY 10020

Copyright © 2002 by Michael Albertson and Ellen Albertson
All rights reserved, including the right of reproduction in whole or in part in any form.

FIRESIDE and colophon are registered trademarks
of Simon & Schuster, Inc.

For information about special discounts for bulk purchases,
please contact Simon & Schuster Special Sales:
1-800-456-6798 or business@simonandschuster.com

Designed by Diane Hobbing of Snap-Haus Graphics

Manufactured in the United States of America

10   9   8   7   6   5   4   3   2   1

Library of Congress Cataloging-in-Publication Data is available.

ISBN 0-7432-2528-7

Temptations is dedicated to our children,
the result of our in-depth, hands-on research.
And to coffee, chocolate, and wine, without which
this book would never have been completed.

{ a c k n o w l e d g m e n t s }

To our agent, Brian DeFiore, for seeing what *Temptations* could be even before it was. A true publishing guru who illuminated the path with his shrewd advice, keen insights, and calming words, all done with unyielding class and supportive laughs (even when the jokes weren't that funny).

Special thanks must go to our editor, Doris Cooper, for "getting it," enthusiastically championing it, sticking with it under trying circumstances, challenging us, and teaching us. We could go on and tell you what a great editor and person Doris is, but we're afraid she'd just tell us to "cut the extra words." So we'll just say: Thank you, Doris.

{ c o n t e n t s }

introduction:
The joy of aphrodisiacs

Ensuring the survival of our species, the quest for food and sex are the most basic human drives. The search for amatory bliss, and the hunt for substances that provide it, are as old as the dawn of civilization. Let's face it, we all want better sex lives.

Lucky for us modern Homo sapiens, we don't have to hunt and forage for aphrodisiacs. Nowadays, sexual stimulation is as close as your pantry or supermarket.

In fact, you've probably eaten aphrodisiacs today. Did you have coffee with a doughnut this morning? A bowl of minestrone with garlic bread for lunch? Perhaps you snacked on a handful of nuts during work or ate chocolate for dessert.

Congratulations, you've consumed aphrodisiacs! See, wasn't that easy? Think of all the fun you could have had if you only knew.

Consider *Temptations* your personal aphrodisiac owner's manual: a culinary road map to romance, love, and lust.

In *Temptations* we'll tell you exactly what foods can turn you and your lover on and how to shift your libido into high gear; and we'll give you ways to revitalize your body with foods that will make you fit for life—especially your sex life.

We'll show you how to identify aphrodisiacs that are scientifically proven and guide you in creating delicious aphrodisiac-laced meals quickly, simply, and easily, so that you have plenty of time and energy for dessert. (Dessert is you!) We have also included foods that are historically purported to enhance sexual performance but have not yet been put through rigorous scientific evaluation. Of course *we* have put them through our own rigorous and energetic evaluation process.

Hey, someone has to do it.

Cooking and eating are like making love. The same senses—smell, sight, taste, hearing, and touch—play key roles in the kitchen and in passion play. Just by cooking a good meal, you are engaging in an erotic act. And unlike shopping in a sex boutique, which can be embarrassing ("Do you have those edible undies in a size 18?") no one needs to know exactly what your plans are for those pine nuts or oysters. What's more, aphrodisiacs and sex are actually good for you. We will reveal the superior nutrients in aphrodisiacs that ward off heart disease, cancer, PMS, and a wide variety of other ailments. Lovemaking itself is a form of healing that is promoted by everyone from Marvin Gaye to heart doc Dean Ornish. Many scientific studies have shown that sex enhances and heals relationships while promoting wellness. New research by Drs. Francis X. Brennan, Jr., and Carl J. Charnetski of Wilkes University suggests that a moderate amount of sexual activity strengthens the body's immune system and fights colds, flu, and other diseases. So it stands to reason that anything that promotes lovemaking can have beneficial effects on your well-being.

Now it's official: Aphrodisiacs are good for your health, too!

From the Dawn of Time to Today

Aphrodisiacs have been part of human existence and the human diet since the beginning of recorded time. African hunters devoured raw lion organs. The Romans preferred wild wolf penis and crocodile semen, and the Egyptians, poisonous serpents. To assure virility on their wedding night, Prussian bridegrooms ate the testicles of wild goat, boar, or bear. Today, tiger penis and rhino horn are still sought-after aphrodisiacs in China. The greatest lovers and most passionate writers throughout history—from Aristotle and Pliny to Shakespeare and Casanova—have seized the power of aphrodisiacs. Leave it to the Bard, who warned in *Macbeth* that alcohol "provokes the desire, but it takes away the performance," to write the perfect example of how aphrodisiacs, if used properly, can enhance pleasure or, used improperly, can fall flat.

It's no coincidence that in modern America, where home-cooked meals are an afterthought, we have one of the highest divorce rates (about 50 percent) of any developed country. In France, the divorce rate is noticeably lower than America's, romance is a way of life, aphrodisiacs grace the plate, and bad food is taboo. Are you starting to see a connection here? Every meal is an occasion to celebrate sensuality and toast love, romance, family, and life. Good food served on a bed of romance leads to a happy, healthy, long, loving, sexually satisfying life.

From Beefcake to cheesecake

Food and sex are intimately entwined in our bodies and minds. Even our language associates food with sex. Just consider the culinary-charged terms used in the game of sexual pursuit—*beefcake, cheesecake, honey, sweetie pie, sugar britches, sugar daddy, buns, sausage, melons, meat,* and *nuts.* (Quite a meal!) In fact, the ancient Greeks were so aware of the food/sex connection that cheesecakes were baked in the shape of a woman's breast, thus linking the taste buds with the libido and inventing one of the greatest desserts in history (or is it herstory?), that eventually gave birth to today's wedding cake.

During World War II, G.I.'s longing for female companionship placed pictures of a scantily clad Betty Grable and her glamorous gams over their beds and referred to the pin-up as "cheesecake." Leggy actresses weren't the only bodies up for show. In the early 1950s erotic photographic displays of the male physique began to be exhibited in bodybuilding magazines. Eventually these pectoral pictorials began filtering into mainstream society and the term *beefcake* was born.

. . .

There are a number of reasons why aphrodisiacs have the power to ignite our senses, capture our imaginations, and fire up our libidos. Aphrodisiacs work on many levels and several factors come into play: chemical, sensory, emotional, romantic, social, and energy factors.

The Chemical Factor

Casanova didn't need a double-blind, placebo-controlled research study sponsored by a giant pharmaceutical conglomerate to know that oysters are an aphrodisiac. He listened to (or perhaps watched) his body respond. Finally, science has explained what he experienced: Oysters are rich in zinc, a male virility mineral. Ol' Casanova knew his stuff. Our sexual organs and endocrine system need special nourishment. Every day he ate dozens of oysters off the breasts of a beautiful woman, usually in a warm tub.

Why do women crave chocolate? Because it's an aphrodisiac, tastes fabulous, and contains magnesium, a mineral that many women crave, particularly before menstruation. Chocolate also contains more than four hundred different chemicals, including phenylethylamine (PEA), an amphetamine-like brain chemical that triggers the sense of euphoria that people experience when they fall in love. Chocolate's seductive combination of fat and sugar increases natural pleasure chemicals produced by the brain called endorphins. And the enticing food also contains the stimulants theobromine and caffeine, which rev up the central nervous system and elevate heart rate and blood pressure. All of these help put us in the "love" mood and enhance sexual performance.

The Aztec king Montezuma drank fifty cups of cocoa before entertaining his harem of six hundred women. (Toga, toga, toga!) How he ever found the time and energy to rule his kingdom is beyond us.

Everyone's reaching for Viagra for a reason, and a lot of it has to do with diet. The over-processed, standard American diet is filled with sugar, calories, and fat, which can cause a significant drop in testosterone levels and increase the risk of erectile dysfunction. (Yes, too many double-pepperoni, sausage, and extra-cheese pizzas can rob you of your manhood. Think about *that* the next time you call Domino's.) The standard American diet lacks key vitamins, such as E (which is needed to make sex hormones and sperm) and the B-complex (which helps increase blood flow to the penis); minerals like zinc and calcium (which helps fight osteoporosis, PMS, and even depression); and essential fats, all of which are needed for your body to be a healthy, functioning, sexually vital machine.

There are dozens of foods that have been shown to reverse the aging process and increase your sexual appetite and capacity. Unlike Viagra, these natural sexual stimulants and body boosters don't have negative side effects like headaches, diarrhea, urinary tract infections, and blue/green-tinted vision. (We know, back in school you used to pay big money to a guy named Chemical Carl for the blue/green-tinted vision.) There are many foods that we'll tell you about that work like Viagra does by boosting levels of a molecule called nitric oxide, which triggers erections.

The Sensory Factor

Babies quickly learn to associate certain tastes and smells with comfort and contentment. As adults, tastes and smells remain a trigger, while romantic love and sex become our comfort and contentment.

Eating is an intimate, sensual, and sensory activity that can stimulate our sexual appetites if the right foods are correctly prepared and consumed. Foods that remind us of sex because of their taste, texture, or appearance are turn-ons: Briny seafood, for example, smells and tastes like sexual juices. Not to mention that seafood is rich in nutrients that help boost hormone levels and enhance sexual function. This shouldn't be shocking or come as a surprise; after all, life on earth originated in the sea. Raw seafood is also sensuous and suggestive because of its fleshy, soft texture. Eat seafood with the hands (think of the lobster scene in the movie *Flashdance* and you'll know what we mean) and the food/sex connection becomes even clearer.

We don't need to tell you what bananas, carrots, asparagus, and figs resemble. Look closely as you take a bite and you may find your mind wandering to thoughts of . . . After all, it doesn't take much. The average male thinks about sex eleven times an hour. Flowers, which are plants' sexual organs, remind us of the budding passion of spring—and let's face it, blossoms resemble a vagina. (Just take a look at a Georgia O'Keeffe painting.)

Buying your lover flowers is a simple gesture that communicates: "I want to make love to you." Why? Sensory memory. Smell is a very primitive sense that penetrates immediately and directly to emotional centers in the brain. Because we have been conditioned to associate flowers with affection, that bunch of long-stem roses is a fragrant reminder that love is on the agenda. We'll tell you a number of ways to use flowers as well as other sweet-smelling botanicals to ignite the senses and stimulate the libido. Henry VIII, who was known for his hearty appetites (food, countries, wives, etc. . . .) liked to munch candied roses, violets, and hawthorn. To get their juices flowing, medieval men and women drank a mixture of flowers and myrtle leaves that had been marinated in wine. In the Hindu religion, after a couple is married they spend their first night together on a bed decorated with flowers. Many popular perfumes are made from flower essence mixed with the scents of wild animals.

The Emotional Factor

From the moment we are born, the first way we interact with the world is through food. Food supports and nurtures us at the most basic level. It's one of life's three primary needs, along with shelter and warmth.

Preparing food for each other is a way to give and receive love. Just as in making love, when someone cooks for you, you feel nurtured, and when you cook for someone else you nurture and take care of them. Emotions manifested by a well-made meal and well-made sex are the same. We feel warm, nurtured, cared for, safe, valued, emotionally secure. In other words, loved! "The way to a man's heart is through his stomach" may be a cliché, but it is true.

Memories, emotions, and the senses are all interconnected. In many instances the emotional and sensory factors interact with each other to create extraordinary reactions.

The sensory aroma of food can evoke powerful emotional and highly charged sexual responses. There's a reason why real estate agents tell sellers to bake bread before potential buyers view their home. (In spite of their reputation, it's not because the agent wants a free meal.) Adults under pressure crave simple foods that evoke feelings of happiness and warmth. While you're examining the bedrooms your olfactory glands are processing the smell of baking bread and your deep emotional center is bombarding you with the message: "Buy this house, it smells good. You will be safe and secure. You will be happy. You and your mate can cuddle up right here and make wonderful love in this marvelous house."

The Romantic Factor

Jewelry, expensive dinners, exotic vacations, luxury cars, and other extravagant gifts are some of the ways that we have been programmed by society's marketing machine to show our love. The hidden message isn't very hidden: If you don't buy, buy, buy she'll say "Bye, bye, bye."

Cooking is a gesture that expresses much more love than slapping down a gold card. It is a purely personal act. Cooking a meal spiked with plenty of aphrodisiacs, dressing up or down for dinner, opening a bottle of wine, lighting candles, and enjoying beautiful music and intimate conversation create an atmosphere for romance that money just can't buy.

According to Dr. Pepper Schwartz, professor of sociology at the University of Washington, an author, and a recognized authority on sexuality, for 90 percent of couples the frequency of lovemaking decreases dramatically after only a short period of time together. Why the lack of lovemaking? People are just too busy, bored, tired, or all three, and sex gets neglected.

Temptations is your prescription for adding creativity to your love life, putting the excitement back in sex, and enticing you to make time for each other. Explore our book and you'll find that making a romantic meal once or twice a week is a sure-fire formula for great sex and enhanced intimacy. By setting a time and date each week with your partner you ensure quality time together. It's exciting to anticipate that date and fun to think about how and with what aphrodisiacs you will seduce each other.

The Social Factor

Throughout history food has been an integral part of romantic social structure. In Sri Lanka, when a woman cooks for a man it means that she has a relationship with him, and she calls him "the one I cook for." In Japan, when a man and woman eat from the same bowl of rice it means that they are a couple. As part of the rituals performed in a Hindu marriage to confirm the engagement, the groom's family gives a verbal promise of marriage and feeds misri (crystalline sugar) to the girl's family. (Eating sweets is considered auspicious by Hindus.) After the Hindu wedding ceremony is over the bride and groom feed each other, signifying that they will take care of each other.

Brides and grooms in ancient cultures wore crowns of wheat to symbolize fertility, and in Rome a thin loaf of bread was broken over the marrying couple's heads, and the crumbs were saved and taken home by the guests as tokens of good luck. And tiered wedding cakes originated in merry ol' England, where the bride and groom kissed over a stack of little cakes.

The Energy Factor

Sex is an exchange of energy between two people, a balance between expansive (male, or yang) and contractive (female, or yin) forces. Particular foods and culinary combinations affect this expansive/contractive cycle and have an impact on our energy levels and sexuality. That's one reason we love balanced, romantic, culinary combinations like champagne (a very expansive food) and caviar (a very contractive food). If the diet is unbalanced and there are too many contractive or expansive foods, sexual energy and performance will suffer.

The types of food you eat have a direct impact on how you feel, act, and perform. A heavy diet that includes lots of dense, contractive foods like meat, sweets, hard cheese, and chips can make you feel sluggish, dry, frustrated, and irritable. A diet that is expansive and contains plenty of vegetables, whole grains, nuts and seeds, and fruit can make you feel relaxed, refreshed, receptive, and creative. Learn to listen to your body and eat foods that bring you into the proper balance. We'll show you how to do this in Chapter 10, "The Cooking Couple's Best Sex Diet."

Aphrodisiacs and Us, Aphrodisiacs and You

Why did we write this book? Because we have found that the best, easiest, healthiest, safest, and most fun way to enhance our love life is with aphrodisiacs.

Whether you've just started dating or have been together for forty years, we all want a better sex life. You may be the best lover in the world, and in a relationship with the most beautiful person on the planet, but unless you make the time to do things that enhance your sexuality the relationship will eventually wither. When you take the time to buy, prepare, and share love foods you automatically make the time to nurture and care for each other.

Now it's time to open your mind, body, and *Temptations* to begin your exploration of the joy of aphrodisiacs. So what are you waiting for? You're gonna love this trip. Turn to Chapter 1 and start fooding around!

1

Neptune's Gift: oysters, the Aphrodisiac King

Lewdly dancing at a midnight ball
We should for hot eryngoes and fat oysters call . . .
For what the drunken dame
(take head or tail), to her 'tis much the same
Who at deep midnight on fat oysters sup.

–Juvenal, Roman satirist, date unknown

Oysters are the hermaphrodites of the animal kingdom, the alchemists of the ocean, and arguably the world's most renowned aphrodisiac. We know, you thought Michael Jackson was the hermaphrodite of the animal kingdom. Wrong, boys and girls, it's the miraculous oyster.

Throughout history oysters have been blamed for shameless and lustful activities, from bacchanal orgies to bisexual shenanigans. Their licentious reputation is well earned in science, folklore, mythology, and the bedroom. It seems like oysters and the amorous dance of desire were made for each other.

Oysters are born in the foam of estuaries and tidal bays, which is why these bivalves are associated with the birth of Aphrodite and Venus, the Greek and Roman goddesses of love. Take a look at Botticelli's *Birth of Venus,* where the naked and *very* well endowed goddess emerges from a seashell. We're surprised that Madonna hasn't ripped off this image yet. But then again, maybe the years are finally catching up.

The world's most famous lover of women and oysters,

oyster ABC'S

Adult oysters breed in the summer. Some species of female lay their eggs directly in the water to be fertilized by sperm, while others retain the eggs in their shells and release the spat (the poetic name for oyster young) after fertilization. After hatching, the spat swarm for several days before attaching themselves to a stable site. Edible varieties of oysters are then ready for harvesting in three to five years.

Of the hundred or so different species of oysters, only about two dozen are eaten. There are four major species: *Crassostrea virginica, Ostrea lurida, Crassostrea gigas,* and *Ostrea edulis.*

Crassostrea virginica are usually two to four inches in length and found in the North Atlantic. Common varieties include Wellfleet, Bluepoint, Pemaquoid, Chesapeake Bay, and Cotuit.

Ostrea lurida (Olympia) are small oysters (under 1½ inches) found on the West Coast and generally farmed on Seattle's Puget Sound.

Crassostrea gigas are large oysters that grow in the Pacific Ocean. Look for Yakima Bay, Kumamoto, Penn Cove, and Golden Mantle varieties.

Ostrea edulis (European flat) are found in Europe; often called belons, these oysters can cost as much as $80 per dozen. (With people paying those prices, you know they must work!)

All edible oysters, regardless of their geographic origin, share the same chemical and aphrodisiac properties.

Casanova, claimed oysters were "a spur to the spirit and to love." He routinely ate fifty oysters for breakfast, often in the bathtub, using a young lady's breasts for plates. He even used oysters for love fun such as "games of the tongue," which he played with two women named Armelline and Emile (later to be known as The Indigo Girls). Oysters were placed on the lips of the lovers and sucked in one by one by other members of the ménage à trois.

On other occasions, Casanova lapped raw oysters from between the girl's breasts. Then he would go lower and . . . well, you get the idea. ("Ah, for true ambrosia the oyster must be dipped in the heavenly sauce of love that only a maiden can provide.")

Back in the days of the Caesars, when gluttony was in vogue and beheadings were fashionable entertainment ("Outstanding form, Aroulious. Let's see another"), the Roman emperor Vitellius would eat as many as a thousand oysters at a time. One of the earliest and most famous bulimics known, good ol' Vitellius tickled his throat with a peacock feather so that he could vomit and make room for more oysters. Now that's mollusk mania.

Doin' the Shuck & Jive

Oysters are tough nuts to crack. Who can blame them? Unable to run or fight back, they keep their shells tightly shut, their only defense against numerous prey—which, besides humans, includes starfish, birds, and the oyster drill, a type of snail that makes a small hole in the oyster's shell and sucks out the oyster with its tongue. (Michael: "Sounds like a girl I once met at a Ramones concert.")

Unfortunately, the fresher the oyster, the harder it is to open. And you always want the very freshest oysters. But there are several tricks to relaxing even the tightest shell. (This is one dame where you don't want a tight fit.) Our favorite is placing oysters in the freezer for about five minutes. This relaxes them and makes the next step, opening them with an oyster knife, much easier.

Other oyster aficionados recommend placing them in a hot oven for a few seconds or immersing them in carbonated water for about five minutes. We've tried all three techniques and like the freezer method best.

Always open oysters right before eating them. The two tools needed for "doing it" (the term that professional shuckers use for
(continued)

opening an oyster) are an oyster knife and something to protect your hands. Oyster shells are extremely sharp and can bite back as you open them. Oyster knives are inexpensive (under $5) and readily available at kitchen supply stores and fish markets. In a pinch, you can use a screwdriver or a church key–style can opener. If using the church key, you will need a knife to loosen the oyster meat from the shell.

To protect your hands, you have two options. For the utilitarians among you, a heavy dish towel will do. If you're into the S&M/Goth look, go for mesh gloves. Very handy for dispensing discipline. Before you begin, you'll also want a platter covered with crushed ice to place the oysters on once they are opened, paper towels (this is messy work), and a bowl for discarded shells.

After assembling your tools, scrub the oysters well with a nylon pad or brush under cold running water.

Now it's time to do battle.

1. Place the cupped, curved part of the oyster's shell in the palm of your hand, remembering to protect your hand with a kitchen towel and/or gloves.

2. Insert your knife into the seam or hinge of the oyster and wriggle the knife back and forth to pry the oyster shells apart.

3. Slide the knife around the edges of the top shell, being careful not to spill any oyster liquid. The delicate nectar of Aphrodite contains tremendous flavor reminiscent of the briny delights below (why do you think they call it "seamen"?) and contributes greatly to oysters' aphrodisiacal effect.

4. Using your knife to loosen the oyster meat from the bottom shell, remove and discard the top shell and any bits of debris or oyster shell that are on the opened oyster, then place the oyster on ice.

5. Serve ASAP with lemon juice, Tabasco sauce, or a dash of caviar. (See The Cooking Couple's Oyster Menu for Amour, page 40, for other serving suggestions.)

Be patient. "Doing it" takes practice.

While most of us are stuck with the gender and genitals God gave us (modern science and several hundred thousand dollars in medical bills notwithstanding), oysters are bisexual bivalves capable of rhythmical hermaphroditism. In other words, they can switch from male to female or vice versa, which they do frequently as the seasons and water temperature change.

Sounds like Elton John at a Versace show.

The Unique Passion Food

No other food smells, tastes, looks, has the texture of, and enhances human sexual response like the oyster.

He who loves without oysters does not truly love.

−Anon., fifteenth century

Why do oysters excite palates and passion? In the case of oysters there is clear chemical and physiological proof to support more than two thousand years of historical, anecdotal, and mythological evidence.

Oysters, often referred to as the "milk of the ocean," are nutritional powerhouses, yet low in fat and calories. (One oyster has about ten calories.) They are packed with the mineral zinc (three ounces contains about 500 percent of the daily requirement), a key element for the production of testosterone, which fuels the sex drive for both men and women.

Zinc is a male virility mineral. A study published in the *Journal of the American Medical Association* found that giving men in their sixties a zinc supplement actually doubled their testosterone levels. (God knows what it would do for the sexual potency of men in their twenties!)

An important component of the male ejaculate, zinc also aids in the proper function of the prostate, which needs ten times more zinc than any other organ in the body. The prostate gland,

oyster trivial pursuit

- King Theodore of Corsica claimed that his three greatest passions were love, military glory, and oysters.
- Oysters were a favorite food of Queen Elizabeth I. (Have you ever seen pictures of this old battle-ax? She needed all the help she could get.)
- For inspiration and sustenance, Mozart was primed with generous amounts of oysters and wine while writing his romantic opera *The Magic Flute.*
- King Henry IV ate so many oysters that they gave him his renowned bellyache. (Most likely it wasn't the oysters' fault. Henry, who had both leprosy and epilepsy, was not well or well liked. There is speculation that the bellyache may have been the result of a poisoning attempt.)
- Louis XIV, whose minimum portion was one hundred, made oysters fashionable at the French court.
- Marshall Turgot, one of Napoleon's officers, ate a hundred oysters each morning for breakfast to give him courage in battle.
- American financier and philanthropist Diamond Jim Brady (aka James Buchanan Brady), known for his opulent lifestyle, love of ostentatious jewelry, and enormous appetite, was so fond of oysters that at New York City's Delmonico's, America's most glamorous restaurant at the time, he once ordered five dozen as an appetizer. (He had two waitresses as his entrée.)

which is located under the bladder, plays a vital role in male sexuality, secreting about 30 percent of seminal fluid (which lubricates and combines with semen) and providing the power to make ejaculation possible. (See "The Cooking Couple's Best Sex Diet," page 279, for more info on the prostate.)

Zinc deficiency in men has been associated with infantilism of the sex organs (ouch!) and loss of sexual potency. Plus, low zinc counts in the bloodstream have been linked to low sperm counts.

You don't need a Ph.D. to add up these numbers, boys. Eat oysters, protect Mr. Happy! Or, as the Oyster Institute of America says, "Eat oysters, love longer!"

Should we also add, "Love bigger"?

In women, zinc increases vaginal lubrication and studies sug-

selecting and storing oysters

Oysters are extremely perishable, so you need to be careful when buying them, especially if you plan to eat them raw. First, when purchasing oysters (or any seafood) go to a reliable seafood market that you trust. Reputable seafood stores must display a government certificate guaranteeing that all seafood sold on the premises (including oysters) have been purchased and handled in accordance with federal guidelines.

If you have a health condition such as cancer or HIV and/or a weak immune system or are pregnant, you should avoid eating raw oysters entirely. Cooking does kill harmful bacteria, so feel free to eat oysters that have been cooked completely. However, cooking also lessens the aphrodisiac effect of oysters, so, as we like to say: Just like good sex, oysters are best au naturel.

There are five things you want to look for when purchasing oysters:

1. Like all bivalves, oysters in the shell must be sold live. Live oysters should feel heavy (which means they are full of juice).
2. Oysters should have a pleasant, fresh, sweet, briny aroma.
3. Oysters should be displayed cup (curved) side down, on top of, *not* buried in, a bed of fresh crushed ice. If they are stored on their sides, they lose juice and spoil faster.
4. Purchase oysters only with intact shells. If the shell is broken, your oyster is dead or dried out.

(continued)

5. Oyster shells should be tightly closed. If an oyster shell is slightly open, tap it. If the oyster is alive, it will close its shell right away. If the shell does not close, the oyster is dead and should be thrown away.

When you get your oysters home, place them curved (cup) side down to prevent liquid from escaping. Store in a shallow bowl, covered by a damp cloth, in the refrigerator. Do not store them in a tightly closed bag or container or in fresh water. Oysters need to breathe.

Their flavor is best within the first twenty-four hours after purchase. We always get our oysters on the day we plan to eat them. Although they will remain alive under refrigeration longer, oysters are best eaten within a week of harvest and no more than three days after you purchase them.

Don't be shy about asking the market when the oysters were harvested. If the answer sounds fishy, fish in other waters.

Shelled oysters, which are used in cooked dishes such as oyster stew or stuffing, are sold canned or frozen and have been pasteurized. While not as flavorful as freshly opened, live oysters, they are convenient. Canned oysters should be used by the expiration date, and once they have been opened, stored in the refrigerator.

Frozen oysters will keep for two to three months and should be defrosted in the refrigerator before use.

gest that a mild zinc deficiency may increase a women's susceptibility to the vaginal fungal infection candidiasis.

Zinc levels decrease prior to menstruation, and women with premenstrual symptoms tend to have lower overall levels of zinc. This leads some scientists to believe that additional zinc may decrease PMS symptoms. (So if your wife, girlfriend, or this summer's fling turns into a character from *Beetlejuice* every third week of the month, try a date at the raw bar.)

Consuming adequate amounts of zinc during pregnancy also

helps ensure the delivery of larger, healthier babies that are carried to term. (Again, pregnant women should not eat raw oysters for their extra zinc.)

Zinc found in oysters is more readily absorbed and used by the body than zinc found in supplements. So get naked and crack those shells.

Nutritionally, oysters are an ideal energizing substance for pre-coitus cuisine or a postcoital refill. These mollusks are high in iron (half a dozen supply a day's requirement), iodine, complex sugars, protein, and the mineral phosphorus, which has been recommended as an aphrodisiac for centuries. (Some old medical texts dealing with aphrodisiacs have even recommended drinking seawater to gain additional phosphorus. The modern American diet provides more than adequate amounts of phosphorus, and deficiency is rarely a problem. While a little extra phosphorus can't hurt, very high intakes can have a negative effect on your calcium stores.) Oysters also contain mucopolysaccharides, gel-like substances made from proteins and sugars that hold body tissues together and work as an aphrodisiac by increasing libido and the production of seminal fluid.

sex in a shell

The American gastronome M. F. K. Fisher, author of fifteen books including *Consider the Oyster* and *Gastronomical Me,* takes a somewhat less scientific view of oysters' erotic qualities: "There are many reasons why an oyster is supposed to have this desirable [aphrodisiac] quality. . . . Most of them are physiological, and have to do with an oyster's odor, its consistency, and probably its strangeness."

Next time you encounter an oyster on the half shell, take a closer look. What do you see?

Oysters resemble human genitals, especially when eaten raw.

Take a sniff. Is that sweet, briny aroma familiar?

oyster cookery

Never overcook oysters unless you like chewing on rubber.

Oysters can be poached, baked, sautéed, fried, and even grilled and should be cooked just until the meat plumps and the edges curl. Smaller oysters are generally more tender and require slightly less cooking time than larger oysters, which can be cut in half before cooking. Cooking oysters in their shells (which can be done with both grilling and baking) will keep the flesh moist and boost the flavor. For a classy presentation, serve cooked oysters in the bottom shell, from which the meat can easily be pried with a fork.

The most famous oyster dish, oysters Rockefeller, was created in 1899 by Jules Alciatore at the world-famous New Orleans restaurant Antoine's. The original recipe, which called for copious amounts of butter, was so rich that it was named for the head of the Standard Oil Company, John D. Rockefeller.

Jules made the dish by baking three dozen oysters in their shells on a bed of rock salt for five minutes. He then topped them with a sauce made from puréed spinach, green onions, parsley, Tabasco sauce, butter, bread crumbs, and sometimes a little absinthe (when it was legal). The oysters were then baked for an additional five minutes.

New Orleans has given birth to several other famous oyster dishes, including oysters Suzette (with pimento and bacon), oysters Catheryn (with artichokes), and oysters O'Hanlon (with onions and eggplant).

Think of the last time you made hot, desperate, animalistic love in an enclosed area. Ah, now you know what we mean.

Oysters' fleshy texture and pleasant, salty flavor exude sexuality. It's as if God took the essence of sexual passion, wrapped it in an almost indestructible jewelry case, and presented the prized trinket to the human race as a gift.

Forget diamonds; *oysters* are a girl's best friend.

. . .

Oysters are not a staple food, like bread, that you mindlessly munch at lunch. Oysters are special. For us, the ultimate romantic offering is a dozen lovingly (and, might we add, painstakingly) opened oysters presented on a bed of ice accompanied by hot sauce or perhaps a dab of caviar, champagne, and a lover clad in something silky, revealing just a hint of what the night will bring.

our oyster pantry

We like to keep a pantry full of different ingredients to top raw or cooked oysters with whatever appeals to us at the moment. Consider the following as accompaniments to complement *raw* oysters:

- Lemon wedges
- Worcestershire sauce
- Tabasco or other hot sauce
- Cocktail sauce
- Mignonette sauce (chopped shallots in red wine vinegar)
- Grated horseradish
- Freshly chopped parsley, chives, or dill
- Thyme, celery seed, or fennel seed
- Cayenne, paprika, or curry powder
- Caviar or salmon roe
- Black Sambuca or other licorice-flavored liqueur
   For complementing *cooked* oysters try:
- Goat or other strong-flavored cheese such as Asiago or Parmesan
- Pesto
- Romesco sauce (a robust Spanish sauce made from peppers, garlic, and nuts)
- Gremolata (2 minced garlic cloves mixed with 1 teaspoon grated lemon peel and ¼ cup chopped parsley)
   To drink with oysters we suggest champagne, dry sherry, Riesling, Sauvignon Blanc, or an oaky Chardonnay.

Oriental oysters, Netherlandish Delight, and Parisian Passion Ammo

Chinese society has been enjoying oysters' arousal power even longer than Westerners. The ancient Chinese cultivated oysters in saltwater ponds as early as 320 B.C. According to Daniel Reid, author of *The Tao of Health, Sex, and Longevity,* oysters were listed in Chinese medicine as an aphrodisiac when eaten fresh and raw, because they contain a number of active hormones and enzymes. According to French marine biologist Arnaud Lacoste, "Oysters, like humans, have a defense mechanism against stress that starts with the secretion of hormones that are the same as those found in humans."

In the tale "The Oysters and the Concubine," a rejected concubine tries to win back her Ming dynasty warlord by secretly feeding him one hundred oysters. That night she sneaks into his bedroom hoping to romance him, but she is too late. He is already vigorously engaging his whole harem. (This story is due to be made into a major motion picture starring Julia Roberts and Chow Yun-Fat, titled *Hidden Oyster, Broken Shell.*)

During Chinese New Year, dried oysters (or *ho xi*) are still eaten to bring all good things in the coming year, because in Cantonese a homonym for oyster, or *houxi,* is "good business."

Of course, oysters have nothing to do with the explosive growth of the Chinese population, right?

Je vis absolument comme une huître. *(I live just like an oyster.)*

—Franz Kafka
(This from the guy who wrote The Metamorphosis.*)*

Oysters, which grow wild throughout the world's oceans—on both coasts of North America and in Europe, Asia, and Australia—are a universal love food. During the seventeenth century in the

oyster mushrooms

For mushroom and mollusk enthusiasts, we have the perfect food: oyster mushrooms. Like their namesake, oyster mushrooms grow in clusters, have a shell-like shape, and are available wild and cultivated. Hailed in a Sung dynasty (A.D. 960–1280) poem as "the mushrooms of flower heaven," oyster mushrooms come in a rainbow of colors, including white, blue, gray, brown, yellow, and pink.

These fungi, like many other types of mushrooms, are also great for your bod. Besides being high in protein and low in calories and fat, oyster mushrooms show promise on the medical frontier. Studies indicate they can improve cholesterol levels and inhibit tumors.

Oyster mushrooms have a velvety texture and delicate, mild flavor that is enhanced by herbs and cream sauces and works well in chicken, veal, pork, and seafood dishes.

The simplest way to fix oyster mushrooms and bring out their flavor is to sauté them in a tablespoon or two of butter or oil with a chopped onion and/or a clove or two of garlic. Oyster mushrooms can also be grilled or added to soups, pasta dishes, stews, and sauces. For a double oyster delight, try our recipe for Simple Sautéed Oysters, page 42, with a side of sautéed oyster mushrooms.

Mushrooms are more than a culinary treat. One of the most popular mushrooms in the world, the shiitake (also known as the Chinese black mushroom), has for centuries been hailed as an aphrodisiac. The ancient Egyptians believed mushrooms were the plant of immortality and declared the fungus fit only for royalty. Mushroom rituals were common in Russia, China, Greece, Rome (Nero called mushrooms "the food of the gods"), Mexico, and Latin America, and the plant was believed to impart superhuman strength and lead the soul to heaven.

Netherlands, oysters were the symbol for all aphrodisiacs. Many Dutch paintings of this so-called golden century depict youths drinking, playing music, courting, and consuming these succulent seducers.

Is it a coincidence that the French, one of the most romantic and gastronomically adept people on the planet, eat more oysters per capita than the citizens of any other country? (The French word for oyster, *huître,* is also slang for "female genitalia.")

In France, oysters are on the plate at every special occasion and on the menu at every good French restaurant. The record for "doing it" (shucking oysters) belongs to Marcel Lesoille, a Frenchman who opened 2,064 oysters in one hour. To the French, the oyster has always been the champion of what the famous gastronome Brillat-Savarin called the *sens genesique,* a "sixth sense" that uses all the senses to bring the sexes together.

Not only are French oysters famous as passion ammo, they were also used by Catholic armies in 1573 as projectiles to rain down upon the Huguenots during the eight-month siege of La Rochelle. (So what was their goal? To make the Huguenots f–k themselves to death?)

Why, then the world's mine oyster, Which I with sword will open.

—william shakespeare, *merry wives of windsor*

when in Rome . . .

In 103 B.C. the Romans began cultivating oysters, the first effort in the West to domesticate wild seafood, in the region of Baia near Naples. Oysters were kept in salt pools, fed wine and pastries, and eaten as an appetizer during many a Roman orgy. (You know what the main course was!)

The Romans introduced oyster cultivation to Britain in 407.

PearL NeckLess?

Don't bother looking for pearls. They are formed in some types of oysters when nacre, the material inside oyster shells, builds up around a piece of foreign matter, such as a grain of sand. The oysters that make these precious spheres are a completely different species from edible oysters.

By the way, the legend of Cleopatra dissolving pearls in vinegar and drinking the liquid as an aphrodisiac is false. She actually used white M&M's. It makes you wonder how Mark Antony conquered anything if he was this easily duped. Apparently, Mr. Antony was thinking with his . . . sword at the time.

Even 1,500 years ago the Romans knew that the Brits needed all the help they could get when it came to sex. It's nice to see that things haven't changed much in merry ol' England after all these years.

He had often eaten oysters, but had never had enough.

–W. S. GILberT of GiLberT & SuLLivan

In Georgian and Victorian London, before the Thames and the North Sea were polluted, oysters were cheap, abundant, and frequently served free in pubs as bar snacks, accompanied by pints of porter. (A classic aphrodisiac balancing act of an expansive food, beer, and a contractive food, oysters. More on this in Chapter 10, "The Cooking Couple's Best Sex Diet.")

Today, microbreweries on the Isle of Man (located in the Irish Sea, between Great Britain and Ireland) still make a traditional oyster stout called Bushy's Oyster Stout by boiling oysters with the beer wort during the brewing process. (Tastes bad, works good.)

Marston's, one of the world's best breweries, also makes a dry, oaky stout designed to complement oysters.

oysters in America: Better Late Than Never

Native Americans on both coasts considered oysters a staple food and left huge piles of shells 2,500 to 3,500 years ago as evidence of their appetites. Wampum, beads of polished shells, were strung on strands, belts, and sashes and used as ornaments and money.

Not to be outdone by their native neighbors, early American settlers devoured ten bushels a year per capita. (A bushel equals thirty-two quarts.) In 1621 the Pilgrims in Plymouth, Massachusetts, served baked oysters on the half shell as part of the first Thanksgiving feast, along with venison, cornbread, homemade wine, and possibly wild turkeys. Oysters were so plentiful that the first colonists of Jamestown described the mollusks that they found in Chesapeake Bay as lying "thicke as stones," and Benjamin Franklin once fed a bucket of oysters to his horse. (That'll put some giddyap in your pony.) You do have to wonder what these "Puritans" did with all that sexual energy.

Oh yeah, they raped, pillaged, and wiped out the Native Americans while remaining chaste and God-fearing.

Could the massive explosion of the American population in the nineteenth century be connected to this oyster bingeing? Not only did oysters help keep early American settlers alive, they helped fuel expansion westward across the Great Plains. Throughout the nineteenth century, raw and cooked oysters were a national passion; people couldn't get enough of the aquatic treat. Annual oyster production in Chesapeake Bay alone was over 111 million pounds, compared with only 4 million pounds in 1990.

Oysters were such an important component of American cuisine that an "Oyster Line" was created to deliver the mollusks via stagecoach to hungry settlers hankering for their fix. Oyster mer-

R is for . . .

One of the most common oyster myths is "Eat oysters only in months that contain the letter *r*." This guideline was written before the days of modern refrigeration, when oysters would spoil quickly—particularly in the warm "r"-less months of May, June, July, and August. Today modern refrigeration has made most oysters a year-round treat.

While summer is the most popular time to enjoy oysters, that's actually when they are the least tasty. Oysters and other shellfish spawn in the warmer weather, and during mating season oysters lose some of their taste and become fatty and soft, as opposed to lean, meaty, and flavorful. If you want to enjoy oysters in the summer, look for ones that have been farmed or imported from cooler waters.

When you go for the raw, stick to oysters from cooler waters and regions such as New England and the Pacific Northwest. The warm southern waters of the Gulf Coast, off the coasts of Alabama, Florida, Louisiana, Mississippi, and Texas—particularly from May through September—so ideal for growing plump, succulent oysters also provide the perfect breeding ground for a potentially deadly type of bacteria called *Vibrio vulnificus.*

chants kept their charges alive by housing them in saltwater tanks and then packing them in barrels filled with wet straw and shipping them across the country by stagecoach, rail, and canal. Before the railroad was built, oysters were rapidly shipped from Baltimore (which today still has some roads paved with oyster shells) to Pittsburgh via stagecoach and ferried downriver to oyster parlors in Cincinnati and other inland cities.

Even honest Abe got in on the oyster orgy. Lincoln was well known back in Illinois for the oyster parties that he held at his home, where oysters were the only thing on the menu. For a man who obviously appreciated the power of oysters, you would think that Abe could have smiled more. But then again, he was married to Mary Todd Lincoln, a woman who could wipe the smile off Bozo's face.

Shortly after the Gold Rush of 1849, Hangtown Fry, one of the most famous American oyster dishes, was created in the California town of Placerville (known back then as Hangtown because it was a major center for administering justice as well as transacting business) at the Cary House by a chef named "Nick Hangtown."

According to legend, a miner who had just struck it rich came into the Cary House Hotel demanding the priciest breakfast available. The expensive dish made from oysters and eggs soon became a San Francisco signature breakfast and a favorite dish for gold diggers working in the mining center. Add a prostitute for dessert (yes, they were in abundance in Hangtown) and the meal could be called Hangtown Fry with cheesecake. The combination of fried eggs and oysters with a side of bacon was also a favorite last meal for condemned prisoners prior to execution.

Who wants to die with their mast at half-staff?

{ Hangtown Fry }

During the California Gold Rush of 1849, meat, eggs, and oysters were extremely expensive foods. Eggs alone sold for about 50 cents each, and oysters and bacon were practically worth their weight in gold, so indulging in a plate of Hangtown Fry cost $6 to $7, a small fortune back then. Today, Hangtown Fry will set you back only a few bucks and makes for a wonderful romantic brunch or two A.M. snack when you're hankering for a little refueling. Here's this quintessentially American dish.

5 large eggs

2 tablespoons milk

1/2 teaspoon salt

Dash of pepper

1/2 cup shucked oysters (cut large ones in half)

Flour

2 tablespoons butter

2 tablespoons chopped parsley

6 strips crisply fried bacon or 4 cooked sausages

1. Break eggs into a small bowl. Add milk, salt, and pepper. Mix with a fork to combine yolks and whites.

2. Dip oysters in flour, covering them completely. Shake off excess. Melt butter in a large frying pan over medium-high heat. Add oysters and cook, stirring oysters to brown evenly, for 1 to 2 minutes.

3. Pour egg/milk mixture into pan. When eggs start to set, lift edges and let uncooked egg flow underneath. When eggs are completely set, loosen omelet with a spatula and flip onto a plate, bottom side up. Sprinkle with parsley and serve with bacon or sausages.

You can also use canned oysters if fresh, shucked ones are not available.

Serves 2

While most of the oyster eateries that were so popular a hundred years ago have disappeared, raw oysters on the half shell are making a comeback in raw bars, upscale seafood restaurants, steakhouses, and the bedroom. Americans eat more than one hundred million pounds a year, both raw and cooked.

To compensate for overharvesting, industrial pollution, oil spills, and red tide, which have made oysters a luxury food, aqua farming and oyster cultivation have taken hold.

A large percentage of today's oyster catch comes from supervised beds. (With the way oysters procreate, someone better supervise those beds.) After the New England beds were depleted oysters were imported from Chesapeake Bay to replenish fished-out oyster beds from Cape Cod to Long Island Sound. First old oyster shells were laid down on the fished-out areas and larvae were shipped in and placed on the old shells to spawn. The baby oysters were then replanted two or three times from bed to bed, where they were allowed to grow to their full size before being harvested.

Oysters are still cultivated in much the same manner, except the water and oysters are tested constantly to make sure the shellfish are safe for consumption.

So whether you crack 'em, shuck 'em, suck 'em, or fry 'em, whether you're eating them from the breast of your beloved or dipped in the golden nectar of love, let Neptune's gift and Aphrodite's surfboard carry you down the carnal rapids of desire to where the gods of passion rule.

As smoothly as these briny brothers (or sisters) slide down your throat, lust will be raising its frisky head from below the waves.

The cooking couple's oyster menu for amour

Here are a few of our favorite quick and easy ways to ignite romance with oysters.

{ oyster shooter }

An aquatic Bloody Mary.

1 freshly shucked oyster

Cocktail sauce

Fresh grated horseradish

Tabasco or other hot sauce

1 ounce plain, lemon-, or jalapeño-flavored vodka

1. Place a freshly shucked oyster in a shot glass. Add cocktail sauce, fresh horseradish, and Tabasco, to taste. Cover with vodka and shoot.

{ baked oysters }

Coarse salt, such as kosher or sea salt

1 dozen live, unshucked oysters, scrubbed

1. Preheat oven to 450° F.

2. Cover the bottom of a baking pan with a bed of salt deep enough to steady oysters.

3. Open oysters, removing the flat top shell and leaving the oysters sitting in their liquid in the cupped bottom shell. Place opened oysters on the bed of salt.

4. Place about 1 tablespoon of selected topping (see Our Oyster Pantry, page 31, for suggestions) on each oyster. Bake in pre-heated oven until hot and bubbly and meat starts to curl slightly, about 8 minutes. Serve immediately.

{ Grilled oysters }

Quick, easy, and festive lazy-man oysters. No shucking required. The oysters pop open on their own.

1 dozen live, unshucked oysters

½ cup of your favorite barbecue sauce or Ginger-Lime Sauce (see below), warmed

1. Preheat grill on high for 10 minutes.

2. Scrub oysters well.

3. Lower grill to medium.

4. Place oysters, cupped side up, directly on the grill grate. Shut grill lid and cook for 3 to 5 minutes, until oysters open slightly.

5. Remove the top shell, and spoon a little barbecue sauce or Ginger-Lime Sauce on cooked oysters and serve right in bottom shell.

{ Ginger-Lime sauce }

1 tablespoon freshly grated ginger root

1 tablespoon sesame oil

2 tablespoons soy sauce

Juice of 1 lime

Whisk together all ingredients in a small bowl. Done!

{ simple sautéed oysters }

Feeling a bit intimidated by "doing it"? Does the thought of eating raw oysters make you feel more queasy than amorous? Here's an easy dish that uses preshucked oysters. Remember, fresh-shucked oysters should always be packed in their own juices, and the oyster liquid should be clear.

Serve with garlic bread and a salad for a completely amorous meal.

2 dozen shucked oysters

½ cup flour

Salt and freshly ground black pepper to taste

2 eggs

½ cup seasoned bread crumbs

2 tablespoons olive oil

1 tablespoon butter

Lemon wedges for garnish

Cocktail sauce

1. Drain oysters and pat dry with paper towels.
2. Season the flour with salt and pepper, and beat the eggs with 2 tablespoons water
3. Dip the oysters, one at a time, in the flour and then the egg followed by the bread crumbs. Set coated oysters aside while you heat the oil and butter. (At this point oysters can also be refrigerated for 2 to 3 hours before cooking.)
4. Heat the oil and butter in a large, heavy skillet over medium-high heat.
5. Sauté oysters, turning once, until oysters are golden brown, about 3 minutes per side.
6. Serve with lemon wedges and cocktail sauce.

Serves 2

oyster aphro-snacks

{ smoked oysters }

Smoked oysters come either refrigerated or canned and make great quick appetizers. Try eating them straight up or on crackers spread with a little cream cheese. You can also make an easy spread by blending the following in a food processor:

8 ounces smoked oysters

16 ounces cream cheese

1 tablespoon fresh dill

1 tablespoon fresh parsley

Salt and pepper to taste

{ angels on horseback }

Traditionally served in Britain after dessert to balance the sweet taste before the port is poured, this recipe is terrific around the clock and a great way to use freshly shucked or canned oysters.

3 thinly sliced pieces of white bread

1 dozen shucked oysters, drained

6 slices bacon, cut in half lengthwise

Toothpicks

1. Preheat oven to 400° F.
2. Cut slices of bread into quarters and toast lightly.
3. Pat oysters dry with a paper towel.
4. Wrap each oyster in half a slice of bacon and secure with a toothpick.
5. Place wrapped oysters on a baking sheet and cook until bacon is crisp, 3 to 4 minutes.
6. Remove toothpicks and serve on toast.

{ Aphro-ROLL }

This recipe is for the more experienced cook who is up to the challenge of tackling sushi. It is similar to a California roll, with smoked oysters substituting for crabmeat.

4 slices nori seaweed

1½ cups prepared sushi rice

1 medium cucumber, peeled, seeded, and sliced into thin strips

1 avocado, peeled and sliced into thin strips

2 dozen smoked oysters

Wasabi and soy sauce

1. Place one sheet of nori on a small bamboo sushi mat. Spread a thin layer, about ⅛-inch thick, of sushi rice on nori, leaving about ¼ inch at the ends uncovered.

2. At one end, lay 3 strips of cucumber, 3 strips of avocado, and 6 smoked oysters. Beginning at the end with the cucumber, avocado, and smoked oysters, carefully roll the seaweed over, using the mat to keep the roll tight. Repeat for remaining 3 sheets of nori.

3. Place rolls seam side down on a cutting board and using a sharp knife, cut the roll into 6 pieces. Serve with wasabi and soy sauce for dipping.

2

Queen Chocolate: The Supreme Aphrodisiac Diva

'Twill make Old women Young and Fresh;
Create New Motions of the flesh,
And cause them long for you know what,
If they but taste of chocolate.

—James Wadsworth, *A History of the Nature and Quality of Chocolate*

Chocolate is the diva of the food world and an aphrodisiacal prima donna. She can be a bitch (to your thighs) or an erotic muse who entrances her subjects with a silken touch and seductive allure. As with all divas, you take chocolate's good with the bad because the good is great!

The *Theobroma cacao* plant, known simply as cacao (As Barbra, Bono, Cher, Mick, Madonna, and Aretha will tell you, you ain't no diva until you need only one name) requires very warm temperatures, humidity, and shade as well as its own personal entourage of midges, the little bugs that pollinate the cacao flowers.

Chemically, culinarilly, and coitally, chocolate is one of the world's most magical and sought-after foods. Chocolate has been revered as "food of the gods" and berated as "food of the devil," used as money, valued as medicine; and most of all, it has been prized as a powerful aphrodisiac.

No other food holds chocolate's appeal or mystery or has such a powerful chemical effect on the brain and body. Although chocolate has unlocked many firmly crossed legs across centuries and continents, science still has not been able to unlock the power and passion of this most mystifying elixir. You can buy chocolate chips, chocolate syrup, chocolate sprinkles, shavings, and frosting but you cannot buy chocolate extract.

It doesn't exist.

Scientists have failed to re-create chocolate's flavor. That's because chocolate is composed of more than a thousand flavor components, many of which cannot be isolated, and more than three hundred chemicals, many of which affect our brain chemistry and mood. There are concoctions referred to as "artificial chocolate"; there are also silicone breast implants.

Like sex, when it comes to chocolate, there is no substitute for the real thing.

What you see before you, my friend, is the result of a lifetime of chocolate. . . .

–Katharine Hepburn,
Academy Award-winning actress

Not only does chocolate contain several neuroactive chemicals that can make you feel good, the perfect combination of sweet and fat found in chocolate (chocolate candy is about 50 percent sugar and 50 percent fat) sparks pleasure centers and the release of endorphins in the brain. Research done on laboratory animals (in other words, freshmen) at the Massachusetts Institute of Technology showed that sweet and fatty foods cause pleasure signals to be released from cells located in a portion of the brain called the hypothalamus. The carbohydrates found in chocolate candy also increase levels of serotonin, a chemical found in the brain that elevates and stabilizes mood.

The fat found in chocolate, cocoa butter, is unique. It is solid at room temperature, softens at around 75° F, and melts at slightly below body temperature. While this is a big problem if you are a chocolate manufacturer looking to sell candy in warm climates, it is ideal for creating a sense of pleasure on the palate. This slow meltdown releases a variety of exotic taste sensations. First the cocoa butter dissolves on the tongue like a silken caress; then the rest of the flavor ingredients flow over the tastebuds. What follows is a cascade of gorgeous flavors across your tongue, sweeping you into chocolate's warm and welcoming bosom.

While understanding how chocolate works is almost as complex as understanding love, we know that several chemicals are responsible for chocolate's alluring power and aphrodisiacal renown. Chocolate is a psychoactive food that affects the central nervous system, making you feel good while putting you in the mood for amour. The most intriguing chemicals in chocolate are anandamide and phenylethylamine. Also produced by the brain naturally, they arouse emotions and stimulate physical sensations.

Anandamide is a neurotransmitter (brain chemical) that is similar to THC (tetrahydrocannabinol), the active ingredient found in marijuana, because it acts on the same brain receptors as marijuana and hashish. Derived from the Sanskrit word for *bliss* (*ananda*), anandamide was discovered in chocolate in 1996 by researchers at the Neurosciences Institute in San Diego. The findings created quite a stir in the media and some chocolate companies, who were concerned that chocolate could be classified as a "drug" and require a warning label from the surgeon general: "Caution: Use of this product may create feelings of euphoria and sexual excitement. Do not operate heavy machinery while using, although heavy petting is permissible."

Fortunately the researchers explained to the Drug Enforcement Agency, the righteous protectors of our brain chemistry, that the findings did not mean that chocolate will get you stoned (unless, of course, you consume it in the form of a hash brownie), only that the discovery partially explains why eating chocolate makes you feel good. "Do you feel good, sir?" "Yes." "Book 'em, Dano!"

Chocolate also contains two other related chemicals: N-oleo-

Here come Da Judge

Believe it or not, a lawyer tried to use chocolate as a defense to clear a client accused of smoking marijuana after he tested positive for cannabis in a routine urine screening. According to the journal *Laboratory of Toxicology, 2000,* the lawyer argued that the accused had eaten a massive amount of chocolate, which mimicked the effect of cannabis, resulting in a positive test. Regrettably, the individual was found guilty. However, he doesn't remember it. Now he gets his anandamide neurotransmitters from the prison canteen.

lethanolamine and N-linoleoylethanolamine. These chemicals work synergistically to increase and extend the euphoria by preventing anandamide from being metabolized by the body. Hence, prolonging the chocolate "high."

Chocolate and Marijuana: Chemical Cousins

Marijuana and chocolate are chemical cousins and erotic soul mates. Both substances are aphrodisiacs that work their magic by stimulating the same receptors in the brain.

From Jamaica to Africa and Asia, *Cannabis sativa* (aka marijuana, weed, pot, hemp, grass, mary jane, bhang, etc. . . .) has a centuries-old global reputation as both a medicine and an aphrodisiac that pre-dates the Drug Enforcement Agency by about 4,000 years.

The oldest recorded medical use of marijuana was made in 2700 B.C. by Shen Nung, the Chinese emperor known as the "wise healer." Marijuana has also been very popular in the Near East, where it is used in Tantric practices and is a common ingredient in Ayurvedic aphrodisiac formulas. Hindus have used marijuana for the last 3,000 years, and its ability to sexually arouse is written about in the original text of *The Thousand and One Nights.* In

Pot Poetry

The Persian text *The Fabulous Feats of the Futtering Freebooters* quoted in *The Cradle of Erotica* by Edwardes & Masters, extols the virtues of hashish as an aphrodisiac.

The member of Abu'l-Haylukh remained
In erection for thirty days, sustained
By smoking hashish.
Abu'l-Hayjeh deflowered in one night
Eighty virgins in a rigid rite,
After smoking hashish.
Felah the Negro did jerk off his yard
For all of a week; hashish kept it up hard.
The Negro Maymum, with opiate,
Without stopping to ejaculate,
Futtered for fifty consecutive days.
Allah bepraise him for having fulfilled
Such a task!
But then, fresh vigor instilled,
Obliged to furnish ten days more—
Making sixty days of coition his score—
He fain went on and finished the chore.
During this ordeal Maymum, in bed,
Smoked what held up his penis head:
Hashish!

"The Tale of the Two Hashish-Eaters," one of the eaters is described as having "a dark and lively zabb (penis), so long that the eye might not carry to the end of it."

The Greek physician Discorides recommended juiced marijuana seeds to heat up the libido, and George Washington, Thomas Jefferson, Henry Thoreau, and William Shakespeare all reputedly used marijuana. You don't think someone could make up *A Midsummer Night's Dream* without a little psychoactive help, do you? Recent excavations at what is believed to be Shakespeare's old home in Devon unearthed pipes that contained marijuana residue.

According to Dr. Burke, President of the American Historical Reference Society and a consultant for the Smithsonian Institute, Washington and Jefferson exchanged their favorite smoking blends. Washington reportedly preferred smoking "the leaves of hemp" to alcohol, and wrote in his diaries that he enjoyed the fragrance of hemp flowers. It seems that Washington and Jefferson were the Cheech and Chong of the founding fathers. (Who do you think added the ". . . pursuit of *happiness*" line to ". . . life, liberty, and . . ."? Good ol' Tommy J. himself.

When George Washington and Ben Franklin were in France raising money for the Revolution, Washington left Franklin to return to Virginia because "I wouldn't miss the hemp harvest at Mount Vernon for all the tea in China." Hemp (marijuana), the number one colonial cash crop, was used to make clothes and paper. In fact, the original draft of the Declaration of Independence was written on hemp paper. The stalks were used in manufacturing, and the leaves, well, no one likes to talk about *that* in connection with the founding fathers. (Or perhaps we should say, the founding dudes.)

In the mid-nineteenth century, marijuana was used to treat menstrual disorders and speed up childbirth. And believe it or not, Louisa May Alcott, the writer of the beloved *Little Women,* once wrote that hashish is an aphrodisiac.

Pot fell from grace in the 1930s when "reefer madness" took hold, largely because of its lusty reputation and supposed ability to incite "deviant" behavior. What the church and our moral overseers at the time meant by "deviant" behavior was having great sex.

Many claims have been made that marijuana prolongs sex and makes you more sensitive to your partner and your own physical responses. Several studies have shown that marijuana does increase sexual pleasure for both men and women. The active ingredient in marijuana, THC, heightens sensory perception, increases relaxation, and produces a feeling of euphoria. Plus, in many cases, people who smoke marijuana assert that it makes them feel as if time has slowed down, so lovemaking seems to, or actually does, last longer.

The city of Amsterdam in the Netherlands is the western hemisphere's marijuana capital. In the "red light district" of Amsterdam, you can openly buy and smoke a veritable cornucopia of pot from around the world. Some "coffeehouses," as marijuana cafés are called, even have elaborate menus listing their exotic offerings. (Nirvana Crystal, Vietnamese Black, Northern Lights, Master Kush, Thai Sativa, Super Silver Haze, Critical Mass, AK47, Cream Sodica, and on and on and on.)

Considering marijuana's aphrodisiac qualities, it shouldn't come as any surprise that Amsterdam is also famous for its legal prostitution. Plus, Amsterdam is also the world's largest stopping port for chocolate, where approximately one-fifth of the world's cocoa supply is unloaded. Pot, chocolate, sex. When was

wanna bite my cheese, big boy?

A recent Baylor College of Medicine study published in *U.S. Journal Proceedings of the National Academy of Sciences* found that THC (the active ingredient in cannabis and marijuana) makes female rats hornier. (Yes, Courtney Love was a test subject.) When researchers dosed female rats with pure THC and placed them in cages with sexually active male rats, the females became significantly more sexually responsive. ("Wanna piece of my cheese, you long-tailed hunk?") THC appears to increase sexual responsiveness by interacting with the female hormone progesterone and the neurotransmitter dopamine, both of which are chemical messengers that influence sexual behavior.

the last time you heard about Holland declaring war on anyone? When was the last time you even heard about Holland being grumpy? When was the last time you heard about someone leaving Amsterdam? They also have terrific art museums, tulips, cleaner canals than Venice, and most folks speak English, too. Plus, they don't hate Americans. What are you waiting for?

The Love Chemical

The most potent love-inducing, mood-altering chemical found in chocolate is an amphetamine-like amino acid called phenylethylamine (or PEA). PEA is a natural brain chemical that stimulates the central nervous system, elevates heart rate and blood pressure, and causes the "high" experienced by lovers.

You know how your heart beats a little faster and you feel a bit light-headed when you know he is meeting you at the airport after the two of you have been separated all week? Or how you literally feel dizzy after a smashing orgasm? That's PEA at work. In fact, in the 1800s, way before anyone knew about phenylethylamine, doctors actually prescribed chocolate as a remedy for jilted lovers.

Studies show that PEA also increases energy, elevates mood, and increases feelings of attraction, excitement, giddiness, and euphoria. PEA increases levels of dopamine, a mood-elevating neurotransmitter needed for sexual arousal and response, in the pleasure centers of the brain.

The "chocolate amphetamine," PEA, was discovered in 1979 by Michael Liebowitz and Donald Klein, a pair of psychopharmacologists who advocate eating chocolate to increase levels of PEA in order to combat depression and mimic the blissful, warm, and fuzzy feelings associated with being in love.

But watch out. Like an overdosed diva, high levels of PEA can cause paranoia in some people, and because PEA dilates blood vessels in the brain, it can also trigger migraine headaches. (This is similar to the effects that marijuana and Barbra Streisand have on some people.)

In addition, chocolate also contains caffeine and another closely related stimulant, theobromine. While the amount of caffeine in chocolate is less than other common caffeinated foods and beverages (5 to 35 mg caffeine in a typical one-ounce bar of dark chocolate compared to 60 to 180 mg caffeine in a five-ounce cup of brewed coffee), the combination of caffeine and theobromine gives you a hearty energy boost. (If you doubt the stimu-

chocolates for sex

According to a survey of nearly a thousand adults conducted by Yankelovich & Partners for the American Boxed Chocolate Manufacturers Association, 18 percent of Americans believe that giving a box of chocolate as a gift will increase their chances of getting sex. Of course, there was a difference in opinion between guys and gals. Twenty-nine percent of the men believed giving boxed chocolate improved their chances of getting sex, while only 8 percent of the women agreed. In the days of the Aztecs things were much simpler. Back then, twelve cocoa beans would buy you a prostitute (and save a lot of time).

In another part of the survey, when asked how they would describe their ideal mate, one-third of men (33 percent) said "creamy," while nearly one out of three women (32 percent) said they'd prefer a "solid" mate. Twenty-eight percent replied "nutty," which makes sense since nuts (the preferred filling of men) along with caramel (the preferred filling of women) are America's favorite fillings.

In addition the survey found that 47 percent, almost half, of all Americans hope that giving boxed chocolate will get them a kiss, and 22 percent believe giving boxed chocolates will get them a date.

lating powers of chocolate, just feed a medium-sized piece to a toddler at bedtime and see what happens.)

If you are not feeling well, if you have not slept, chocolate will revive you. But you have no chocolate! I think of that again and again! My dear, how will you ever manage?

–marquise de sévigné, February 11, 1677

Studies show that people crave chocolate more than any other food. Many women will tell you that the desire for chocolate is especially intense between ovulation and menstruation when the hormone progesterone increases the desire for high-fat foods. In addition, premenstrual tension is linked to magnesium deficiency, and chocolate contains magnesium. According to a review of chocolate cravings published in the *Journal of the American Dietetic Association,* a combination of chocolate's sensory characteristics, nutrient composition, and psychoactive ingredients, compounded with monthly hormonal fluctuations and mood

The Truth about chocolate and your Health

People who habitually drink chocolate enjoy unvarying health and are least attacked by a host of little illnesses which can destroy the true joy of living.

–Brillat-savarin, famous nineteenth-century French gastronome and food writer

Chocolate has been blamed for everything from acne to tooth decay. The good news is that in moderation chocolate will not harm your health or complexion and is actually good for you. Here are the sweet facts.

- Chocolate does not cause acne. Two studies—one by the Pennsylvania School of Medicine and another by the U.S. Naval Academy—showed that eating chocolate did not aggravate or cause acne.
- Chocolate does not promote tooth decay. While the sugar in chocolate, as in any other sweet food, can lead to cavities, the cocoa butter in chocolate actually coats the teeth and protects them from plaque formation.
- Chocolate is heart healthy. While the cocoa butter in chocolate is high in saturated fat (the type of fat that can increase cholesterol levels), chocolate contains a unique type of fat called stearic acid. The body turns stearic acid into oleic acid, a type of heart-healthy monounsaturated fat naturally found in olive oil.

  In addition, researchers at the University of California, Davis, have found that chocolate, especially dark chocolate, is a great source of antioxidants called phenolics (plant chemicals also found in coffee, tea, and wine) that can lower your risk of heart disease.
- Chocolate is a good source of iron, magnesium, and copper. Milk chocolate is a good source of calcium.

(continued)

> •In moderation, chocolate isn't fattening. One piece of gourmet boxed chocolate contains about 75 calories, a mini chocolate bar has about 50, and a Hershey's Kiss contains a mere 25 calories.
>
> Although it contains caffeine, the amounts are low enough (5 to 35 mg per ounce) that chocolate is not physically addictive. However, whether it is psychologically addictive is a whole other story.

swings among women, is probably most responsible for female chocolate cravings.

A short, sweet History of chocolate

The superiority of chocolate [hot chocolate], both for health and nourishment, will soon give it the same preference over tea and coffee in America which it has in Spain. . . .

–Thomas Jefferson,
in a Letter to John Adams, 1785

once upon a Time in Meso-America

The first people to discover cacao beans and use them for a beverage were the Olmec civilization, an ancient Meso-American empire living more than 3,000 years ago in the hot, humid lowlands along the Gulf Coast in what are now the southern Mexican states of Veracruz and Tabasco. The Olmec passed their chocolate legacy to the Maya, who migrated from Guatemala to the Yucatan peninsula in Mexico around A.D. 600 and established large cacao plantations.

The Maya and Aztecs crushed cacao beans and mixed them with chile peppers, vanilla, maize, herbs, flowers, black pepper, allspice, annato (which tinted the chocolate bloodred), and water to make a frothy bitter beverage with stimulating and restorative properties. The Maya preferred to drink their chocolate hot, the Aztecs at room temperature (shaken, not stirred). The beverage was consumed after meals, and was called *xocoatl* by the Mayans and *cacahautl* by the Aztecs, both of which mean "bitter water" and may have been the origin of our word *chocolate.* The word *chocolate* might also have come from the native Mexican words *choco* ("foam") and *atl* ("water").

"can you spare a dime? I mean a cacao bean?"

The cacao bean was so valuable to Mayan and other Central American peoples that it was used as money. Ten beans would buy a rabbit, twelve would get you a session with a prostitute, and one hundred would buy a slave. Mayan dignitaries were buried with bowls and jars inscribed with the word *cacao* for making chocolate in the afterlife. (Why go to heaven if you can't have chocolate?) The Maya even had trouble with cacao bean counterfeiters who filled hollowed out beans with dirt. (Could this be the beginning of the famous Chocolate Mud Pie?)

Fill'er up

Chocolate was considered a sexual stimulant by both men and women, and the Aztecs drank it to honor Xochiquetzal, their Aphrodite, or goddess of love. Emperor Montezuma is said to have drunk fifty goblets a day before entering his harem of more than six hundred women. "I would need sixty goblets." "Actually, sixty-five, Michael. You're not nineteen anymore."

white man gets first taste of black ambrosia

Christopher Columbus was the first European to come into contact with chocolate, in 1502, on his fourth voyage to the New World. When he brought cacao beans back to Europe, folks in

That oL' Time ReLigion

In a rite similar to baptism, newborns were anointed with chocolate on the fingers, toes, forehead, and face. Cacao cotillions were a big hit among the Aztecs as a way to display wealth and power and appease the gods. One ritual celebrating the chocolate harvest ended with the presentation of two thousand cups of cocoa served in gold goblets by naked virgins to the emperor and his court. (Hey, who brought the cherries?)

Spain paid little attention to the strange dark beans, as they were upstaged by other treasures such as live Indians, exotic animals, and picture postcards of Disneyland.

Hernando Cortez made it to the New World via Mexico in 1519. The Aztecs there mistook him for the god Quetzalcoatl who, according to legend, brought the cacao tree from Paradise to earth on a ray of the morning star and taught the people how to transform the beans into "ambrosia of the gods," a drink that bestowed wisdom, stamina, and erotic pleasure.

Cortez brought the recipe for chocolate back to King Charles I of Spain. Chuck liked the new drink so much that he ordered Spanish monks to improve the beverage, which they did by adding sugar, cinnamon, vanilla, powdered roses, orange water, almonds, and hazelnuts. The secret of making chocolate was closely guarded from the rest of Europe, and the Spanish cacao monopoly lasted for decades.

A StimuLating Taste of The New worLd

Recognizing the value of cacao beans, or "black almonds," Spain set up the first cacao plantation in the New World. In 1585 the first commercially grown shipment of cacao beans made it back to the Old World. Chocolate was the first stimulating beverage introduced to Europe. (Tea did not arrive until 1610, coffee in 1615.) Imagine, no coffee or tea in the morning. No wonder there was the Hundred Years War in Europe. Everyone was permanently grumpy.

Until the arrival of chocolate, there were no extravagant desserts or sweets. Chocolate was a thick, rich, sweet, and satisfying new taste sensation that captured the taste buds and libidos of the luxury-seeking rich and never let go.

Soon the Eurotrash of the seventeenth century learned what the Aztecs and Mayans already knew and started using chocolate as a love potion for both men and women that would not only enhance romance but was believed to actually "heal" a broken heart.

next stop, italy

By the seventeenth century chocolate was enjoyed by the Spanish royal court, which became famous for its chocolate drinks. Chocolate was introduced to Italy in 1606. Italians were the first people to use chocolate to flavor sweet and savory dishes. In Italy, chocolate gained additional notoriety for its reputation as a vehicle for poison. Pope Clement XIV, who suppressed the chocolate-loving jolly Jesuits in 1773, was believed to have eaten poison hidden in a bowl of chocolate. Moral: Don't mess with the Jesuits.

Bonjour, madame chocolate

Chocolate reached France in 1615 when Anne of Austria, a member of the Spanish royal family, married Louis XIII, king of France. The French court embraced chocolate after the Paris Faculty of Medicine approved it as a "beneficial potion." Drinking chocolate at Versailles with the Royal Court was *the* in thing to do, and by the middle of the seventeenth century chocolate drinking was the height of fashion among French aristocracy. The French court quickly made the chocolate aphrodisiac connection by nibbling on chocolates covered in catherides, a sexual stimulant used in the eighteenth century made from the blister beetle, aka Spanish Fly. Spanish Fly is extremely toxic and in large doses can kill. It contains a chemical called cantharidin that irritates the urinary tract, resulting in increased blood flow and burning sensation in the genitals. Take it from us, there are much better and safer ways to increase blood flow to the genitals.

party poopers

Chocolate is so stimulating and so much fun that you just knew the Church would try to step in and ruin the party. From its beginnings well into the eighteenth century, chocolate was proclaimed by the clergy as "immoral and provocative of immorality," which only made it more popular among the nobility due to its powerful effects. In seventeenth-century France, monks were forbidden to drink chocolate because of its reputed amorous properties. Ever faithful to their reputation as snobby contrarians, the French simply ignored these edicts.

The chocolate made me do it!

While chocolate was esteemed for its medical and aphrodisiacal properties, occasionally it was blamed for some strange side effects. According to the letters of Marquise de Sévigné, a member of the court of Versailles, "The Marquise de Coetloghon took so much chocolate being pregnant last year that she was brought to bed of a little boy who was black as the Devil." Sacre blu. When questioned, Dennis Rodman responded: "Yeah, it coulda been me. . . ."

God save the Queen

Chocolate drinking was introduced to London in 1657 by a Frenchman (You didn't think the Brits would figure out about chocolate's amatory qualities on their own, did you?) who opened a chocolate house where the beverage was advertised as "an excellent West India drink which cures and preserves the body of many diseases." It was a big hit with the wealthy and quickly become chic among the British upper crust. Soon chocolate houses began springing up across London, becoming fashionable places to meet, greet, and plot deceit.

In 1776 there was some little thing going on in "the colonies," but the British were too busy to pay those "irritating rabble-rousers" much notice. The British Parliament was wrestling with important issues like whether to lower the tax on chocolate. They eventually succeeded in doing so, and the lower prices they brought about made chocolate accessible to the general public for the first time. Oh yeah, "the colonies" became known as the United States of America, and England became known as the home of the Beatles, warm beer, and bad oral hygiene.

"I went to a garden party . . ."

According to Moreau of Tours, the Marquis de Sade gave a ball in 1772 where he served chocolate pastilles spiked with Spanish Fly. The result? "All at once the guests, both men and women, were seized with a burning sensation of lustful ardor; the cavaliers attacked the ladies without concealment." Apparently Moreau of Tours was too preoccupied to complete his chronicle of the evening's fun and games. Another guest, Louis Petit de Bachaumont, wrote of the evening: "Into the dessert he [Sade] slipped chocolate pastilles so good that no one failed to eat some. It proved to be so potent that those who ate the pastilles began to burn with unchaste ardor and to carry on as if in the grip of the most amorous frenzy."

Chocolate Goes Modern

Toward the end of the eighteenth century chocolate was enjoyed as a flavoring in ice creams, sorbets, and other desserts, as well as some entrées. In the nineteenth century, technological advances on the chocolate frontier made chocolate cheaper and more versatile. In 1828 Coenraad Van Houten of the Netherlands invented the cocoa press, which removed about two-thirds of the cocoa butter, resulting in a refined cocoa powder that was milder, darker, and mixed better with liquids. The invention decreased the cost of both buying and making chocolate.

The chocolate bar was invented in England in 1847 by J.S. Fry & Sons when chemists at the company learned to remove fat from cocoa beans and mix the remaining cocoa butter with sugar into a thin paste, then mold it into bars. The creamy smooth chocolate quickly became more popular than the old, coarse-grained version.

MOO

In 1876, after eight years of experimentation, Swiss inventor Daniel Peter created milk chocolate and began to sell it. Cows went on strike in protest.

Smooth Moves

In 1879 Swiss chocolate-maker Rodolphe Lindt developed a method of mixing liquid chocolate called conching, which results in a smooth eating chocolate that melts in the mouth.

Jules Séchaud introduced filled chocolates in Switzerland in 1913. In fact, the Swiss eat more chocolate per capita (over 22 pounds per year) than any other country.

Little Beans Become Big Business

In 1894 American candy-maker Milton Hershey began producing candy bars, baking chocolate, and cocoa. Then in 1900 he introduced his milk chocolate bar. Just two years later, construction began on a large factory and town to house his employees: Hershey, Pennsylvania. And the rest, as they say, is very sweet history.

Frank and Ethel, a husband and wife business team, started a little concern in Tacoma, Washington, around 1911. No one paid them much attention until 1923 when Mr. & Mrs. Mars invented the Milky Way bar, which proved immensely popular and was followed by the Snickers bar in 1930.

Ride, ride, ride, Let her ride

In 1926 Lady Godiva arrived on the chocolate scene, riding the growing demand for "luxury" chocolates. Godiva chocolates got their name from the owner's wife, who suggested naming their new products after Lady Godiva, whose legendary exploits (and body) made her famous (or infamous, depending on your morals or lack thereof) throughout Europe.

What Does M&M Stand For?

No, it's not Mickey Mouse. These great little candies that have been an American snacking favorite for decades began life as the offspring of two chocolate behemoth offsprings. Forrest Mars (son of Frank) and Bruce Murrie (son of the president of the Hershey Chocolate Company) founded M&M Ltd. in 1941 and stamped their initials, M&M (Mars & Murrie), on their overnight sensation. A nice way of avoiding an argument over whose name goes first.

Let It Flow

Liquified chocolate was perfected by The Wilber Chocolate Company in 1951 and made deliveries of their chocolate by tanker truck possible. This simplified manufacturing, but unforeseen problems developed when chocoholics attempted to attach feeder nozzles to their faces.

It's not that chocolates are a substitute for love. Love is a substitute for chocolate.

–Miranda Ingram

From a Tree to Your Libido

Chocolate comes from the seeds of a tropical tree botanically known as *Theobroma cacao,* generally called cacao. Chocolate lover and eighteenth-century Swedish botanist Linnaeus named the tree Theobroma, which is Greek for "food of the gods." The amazing *Theobroma cacao* is actually an evergreen tree that reaches a height of 20 to 40 feet and sprouts about thirty giant red or yellow oval-shaped pods a year directly from its trunk. Inside each pod are twenty to fifty cacao beans (the source of chocolate) known to natives as "pepe de oro" or "seeds of gold," aptly named for the powerful and blissful stimulant that lies within their colorful husks. The tree originated in the region between southern Mexico and the northern Amazon basin, and today is cultivated within 10 to 20 degrees of the equator in Africa, Hawaii, the Caribbean, the South Seas, and South America.

While the tree produces fruit 24/7, the pods are harvested only twice a year. After the ripe pods are picked and broken open, the beans are removed along with their surrounding pulp, covered, and allowed to ferment, which develops the chocolate's flavor.

After fermentation, the beans are dried in the sun and sent to chocolate manufacturers, where they are cleaned, blended (there are over thirty different varieties of beans), roasted, skinned, and crushed into chocolate liquor. The chocolate liquor (a misleading term because the chocolate contains no alcohol and is only a liquid when heated) is either defatted and made into cocoa or becomes unsweetened chocolate, the essential ingredient for chocolate confections. Sugar, flavorings (the most common of which is vanilla, but mint, orange, and coffee are also added), lecithin and additional cocoa butter are added to the unsweetened chocolate and then the mixture undergoes conching, which develops the desired chocolate flavor.

Next, the chocolate is tempered (a heating and cooling process that helps stabilize the cocoa butter) and molded into bars or candies.

chocolate's culinary cousin: vanilla, the heaven-scent aphrodisiac

Reminiscent of mother's milk and melted ice cream, at first blush, vanilla appears to be the most innocent of aphrodisiacs. Don't be fooled. Equally appealing to both sexes, vanilla is about as innocent as Lolita. Beneath that comforting, sweet, virginal scent lurks an arousing aroma waiting to engulf you and your lover with its erotic aura.

Vanilla is ranked as one of the five most attractive aromas to men. According to Paris perfumer Jean Paul Guerlin, "There are certain body odors which are very attractive to men and women. All our successful perfumes have two notes: vanilla and an animal scent. In short, they are aphrodisiacs."

According to Tatonic legend, vanilla was born as a love offering. Xanat, the beautiful daughter of the fertility goddess, visited earth and fell in love with a mortal youth. Unable to marry him because he was mortal (not to mention a drummer in an R&R band,

A Drop or Two Will Do

Vanilla is a wonderful external aphrodisiac. In the early twentieth century women dabbed vanilla extract behind their ears as a magical love perfume to attract men. It works. Try some of these:
•Dab a drop on your pulse points before a rendezvous. Your intended's pulses will race to the beat of this tropical spice.
•Draw a bath for two scented with real vanilla extract.
•Mix an ounce or two of rubbing alcohol with the essential oil of vanilla in an atomizer and spritz on like perfume.

which really pissed off Dad), she turned herself into a vanilla orchid so she could belong to her love forever.

Vanilla is the only orchid that is regularly used for food. Like chocolate, it originated in Central America where it still grows wild on the edge of the Mexican rain forest. Today most vanilla comes from Madagascar, the Comoro Islands, and Réunion. The Aztecs frequently added vanilla to their chocolate drinks to enhance the taste and aphrodisiacal power. Vanilla, like chocolate, came to Europe via Spain in the late 1500s. Real vanilla and vanillin, artificial vanilla extract, are still commonly added to chocolate today.

Vanilla quickly caught the aphrodisiacal eye of Elizabethan sybarites due to the vanilla pod's resemblance to a vagina. Elizabeth I, the virgin queen, whose apothecary recommended the spice, boosted its popularity by using it to flavor her marzipan as well as her boudoir. Brillat-Savarin, the famous French writer and gastronome, recommended an aphrodisiacal dish called "pyramid of vanilla and rose meringues." Along with chocolate, the Comtesse du Barry incorporated vanilla into her aphrodisiac arsenal to keep her lovers attentive.

what's in a name?

The word *vanilla* comes from the Spanish word *vainilla,* which is similar to the Spanish word *vaina,* which means vagina.

Because of its legendary creation and its attractive taste and
smell, vanilla has a reputation as a magical food commonly used
to expand love and lust. Food flavored with real vanilla (artificial
vanilla extract lacks the pure, spicy flavor of real extract and has
no magical love power), from ice cream to pudding, can increase
libido and enhance sex. Here are a couple of simple ways to har-
ness the amorous power of vanilla.

·*Vanilla sugar:* Split a whole vanilla bean in half lengthwise.
Place the two pieces in a long jar. Fill the jar with a cup or two of
sugar, close tightly, and let it sit until the sugar has absorbed the
essence of the vanilla. This will take about a week. Then sprinkle
the vanilla-flavored sugar on other love foods such as berries or
freshly whipped cream. Add more sugar to the jar as you use it
and your vanilla bean will continue to spark your food and love
life for up to a year.

·*Vanilla brandy:* Split two vanilla beans and add them to a pint
of brandy, letting the vanilla flavor the alcohol for about two
weeks. This is a great third-date, after-dinner drink that really
gets the party off on the right foot.

Vanilla is powerful and should be used with some caution, as it
can be toxic in large doses. Never use more than two whole beans
at a time in a recipe.

No Energy Shortage Here

Chocolate is the tastiest source of calories on the planet. One chocolate chip provides enough energy to walk 150 feet, thirty-five chocolate chips provide enough fuel to walk about a mile. Depending on how energetic you like your sex, an average romp between the sheets burns about 100 calories. That's four Hershey Kisses, thirty-five chocolate chips, or two tablespoons of chocolate syrup. Plus, an ounce of baking chocolate contains 10 percent of your RDA for iron.

Today the world reveres and celebrates chocolate's undeniable erotic appeal regardless of political, social, geographical, or religious differences. Chocolate has been described as irresistible, naughty, nice, a devilish drug, divine food, illegal or immoral, capable of packing on pounds or pumping up pleasure, erotic, and exotic. In its long history chocolate has been accused of all of these and more for good reason. It's all true!

In our experience the road to a sweeter love life is paved with kisses, truffles, M&M's, ganache, fudge, fondant, hot cocoa, devil's food cake, mousse, haystacks, turtles, mud pie, and Goo Goo Clusters. Ahhhhhhh . . .

All I really need is love, but a little chocolate now and then doesn't hurt.

—Lucy, from "Peanuts" by Charles M. Schultz

Who are we to argue with a diva?

The cooking couple™ chocolate menu for amour

If chocolate is your downfall, you might as well enjoy the trip.

–Godiva chocolatier

{ chocolate bread }

No time to bake? Nonsense. Just pick up an order of uncooked pizza dough at your local pizzeria or supermarket, sprinkle it with a few aphrodisiacs, bake, and say you made the bread from scratch.

1 cup (6 ounces) semisweet chocolate chips

¼ cup cocoa

¼ cup sugar

1 teaspoon cinnamon

1½ teaspoons cardamom

½ cup walnuts, chopped

½ cup raisins

1 order pizza dough (enough to make one large pizza)

1. Preheat oven to 350° F.
2. In a medium-sized bowl combine chocolate chips, cocoa, sugar, cinnamon, cardamom, walnuts, and raisins.
3. Stretch pizza dough out into a rectangle that measures approximately 10x15 inches.
4. Sprinkle stretched dough with chocolate chip mixture.
5. Roll dough into a log, starting at long end. Using a chef's knife, cut a few slits, about 1-inch deep, in the top of the bread. Place on greased cookie sheet and bake until golden brown, about 30 minutes.

{ chocolate banana spring rolls }

Eat these as an appetizer, and you just might become the entrée!

1 medium banana

4 square spring roll wrappers*

¼ cup semisweet chocolate chips

1 large egg, beaten with ¼ cup water added

Vegetable oil for frying

Cocoa for dusting

Chocolate sauce for dipping

Vanilla or coconut ice cream (optional)

1. Cut banana into quarters. (Cut in half lengthwise and then again in half crosswise.)

2. Lay out 1 spring roll wrapper. Place 1 banana quarter and 1 tablespoon chocolate chips on wrapper. Fold right and left sides of wrapper toward center and then roll up cigar-style. Brush with egg/water mixture to seal.

3. Pour 2 inches of oil in a large sauté pan or deep fryer. Heat oil to 350°F. (To test oil, toss in a cube of bread, which will sizzle and brown quickly when oil is hot enough.) Fry spring rolls until golden brown, turning once, about 1 minute per side.

4. With a slotted spoon, remove spring rolls from oil and drain on paper towels.

5. Dust with cocoa and serve with chocolate sauce and ice cream.

Spring roll wrappers are available in Asian specialty markets, and are also carried by some supermarkets.

Serves 4

{ chocolate soup }

This simple recipe for chocolate soup can be varied in a number of ways. For suggestions, see The Chocolate Pantry, page 72.

1 cup chocolate milk

½ cup heavy cream

4 ounces (⅔ cup) semisweet chocolate chips

1. In a double boiler, heat chocolate milk and cream, stirring occasionally, until very hot. Add chocolate chips and heat, stirring frequently, until melted.

2. To serve, ladle soup into bowls and garnish as desired.

Serves 2

{ chocoLate Fruit saLad }

½ loaf chewy French bread, cubed
1 banana, sliced into rounds
2 kiwis, cubed
1 cup fresh berries
1 tablespoon cocoa
4 fresh mint sprigs, to use as garnish

Combine the bread, banana, kiwis, and berries. Using a sieve, sprinkle cocoa on top. Toss, and serve immediately garnished with mint sprigs.

Serves 4

{ chicken MoLe (chicken with chocoLate sauce) }

Mole is a rich Mexican sauce made with spices and unsweetened chocolate. This recipe also works well with sautéed turkey tenderloin. Moles are traditionally served with hot corn tortillas, but can also be served with rice.

2 skinless boneless chicken breast halves, or 2 boneless thighs
3 teaspoons chili powder
2 tablespoons vegetable oil
1 medium onion, chopped
2 cloves garlic, chopped
½ teaspoon ground cumin
¼ teaspoon ground cinnamon
1 (16-ounce) can stewed whole tomatoes, with juices
½ ounce unsweetened chocolate, preferably Mexican,
   chopped
2 tablespoons toasted pumpkin seeds, optional
Salt and freshly ground black pepper to taste

1. Sprinkle chicken with salt, pepper, and 1 teaspoon chili powder. Heat 1 tablespoon of oil in a large sauté pan over medium-high heat. Sauté chicken until brown, about 2 minutes per side. Place chicken on plate and cover to keep warm.

2. Add another tablespoon of oil to sauté pan over medium heat. Add onions and cook until golden brown, about 10 minutes. Add garlic, remaining 2 teaspoons chili powder, cumin, and cinnamon. Cook for 1 minute. Add tomatoes, bring to a simmer, and cook, stirring frequently, until sauce thickens, about 10 minutes. Add chocolate and stir until melted.

3. In a blender or food processor, grind the pumpkin seeds into a fine powder. Add the cooked sauce and blend until smooth. Taste sauce and adjust seasonings.

4. Pour sauce back into sauté pan. Add chicken to sauté pan and cook over medium heat for another 5 minutes.

Serves 2

The Chocolate Pantry

Once you master our recipes for Chocolate Soup and Chocolate Fondue, it's time to experiment with flavorings, dips, and garnishes. Here are some suggestions to get you started. We like to serve the soup or fondue along with extras and let people create their own chocolate fantasies.

Flavorings for fondue or soup

•Several drops of vanilla or almond extract
•A splash of liquor such as crème de cacao, Kirsch, cointreau, Amaretto, brandy, cognac, or spiced rum
•1 teaspoon instant espresso powder

For dipping in fondue or serving with soup

•Bite-sized banana chunks
•Marshmallows
•Toasted pound cake (cut in cubes) or lady fingers

For dipping in fondue

·Strawberries
·Crystallized ginger
·Dried fruit
·Nuts
·Graham crackers

For garnishing soup

·Toasted coconut
·Slivered or sliced almonds, toasted
·Angel food cake
·Whipped cream
·Cocoa
·Nutmeg
·Cinnamon (sticks or powdered)

chocolate Aphro-snacks

{ chocolate fudge sauce }

In a small heavy saucepan heat ½ cup heavy cream with 1 tablespoon butter over medium-low heat, until butter is melted and cream is hot. (Do not boil.) Remove pan from heat and add 6 ounces semisweet chocolate chips (1 cup) and ½ teaspoon vanilla extract. Stir until chocolate is melted.

{ chocolate-covered pretzels }

Melt 6 ounces (1 cup) chocolate chips over a double boiler or in the microwave. Dunk pretzel rods or nuggets in melted chocolate and roll in sprinkles. Set on wax paper to cool.

{ chocolate fondue }

In a heavy saucepan warm ½ cup cream over medium-low heat. (Do not boil.) Add 9 ounces semisweet chocolate chips (1½ cups) and cook, stirring constantly, until chocolate is melted. Transfer to fondue pot and use for dipping fruit, nuts, and cake.

{ Easy chocolate ice cream soda }

In a tall glass mix ½ cup milk with 2 tablespoons chocolate syrup. Add ¾ cup soda water. Stir and top with chocolate, coffee, or vanilla ice cream.

{ chocolate Date shake for Two }

In a martini shaker mix 1½ cups milk with 2 shots coffee liqueur, 4 tablespoons chocolate syrup, and ice. Shake well, strain, and pour into glasses.

{ chocolate chip pancakes }

Stir 6 ounces of chocolate chips (½ cup) into a batch of your favorite pancake batter before cooking. Serve with ice cream and/or chocolate syrup.

3

Princess Aphrodite: Fishing for Love in All the Right Places

Those who live almost entirely on shellfish and fish . . . are more ardent in love than all others.

−Dr. Nicholas Venette in
Tableau de L'Amour Conjugal

Aphrodisiacs are named for Aphrodite, Eros's (aka Cupid's) mother. Perched on her seashell throne, she blesses foods of the sea, casting her powers to stoke lust and bestow pleasure.

Greek gods and goddesses always make dramatic entrances. (Gods aren't born, they arrive.) Aphrodite is no different. In fact, Aphrodite's entrance puts her right on the cutting edge.

The goddess of love sprang from the severed penis of Uranus, the sky god. (Now *that's* a real conversation stopper on the cocktail party circuit: "I'm sorry. I must have misheard you. Where did you say you were from?") Uranus's son, Kronos, in an effort to take over the throne, killed and castrated his father and threw Dad's dick into the sea. The immortal flesh spread into a circle of white foam and from this froth, the goddess of love was born.

"Oh, you're from Froth? That's in Serbia, right? You wouldn't know the Kronos family, would you? Very nice people. They're in the sausage business."

Aphrodite literally means foam-born. And thanks to Aphrodite's blessings, a plethora of sea fare are powerful sexual stimulants.

Seafood has long been linked to love and sex.

•In China, where fish symbolizes regeneration, abundance, prosperity, and connubial bliss, a pair of fish is given to a newly married couple to bless their sexual union.

•Fish were frequently used in Europe in connection with dating and marriage rites.

•A popular Victorian folk ritual called for eating a raw or roasted salt herring on Halloween night and going directly to bed, fish breath and all. The man or woman the herring eater was destined to marry would then appear in his or her dreams with a glass of water to quench the dreamer's thirst.

seafood, sexfood, good food

Fish really have the property of bringing the spermatic secretion into activity.

–Dr. Jacobus X in *The Genital Laws*

There is an ocean of scientific information to back up seafood's reputation as a romance enhancer and health food. What can seafood do for you?

Increases your sexual vitality: Seafood is rich in nutrients, including omega-3 fatty acids, zinc, iron, calcium, and high-quality protein, that fuel sexual vitality and improve overall health.

Fishy Laws

It is illegal in Minnesota for a man to have intercourse with a live fish. (Was this practice so common in Minnesota that they had to pass a law to stop it?) Across state lines in Oblong, Illinois, there is a law that allows newlyweds to be punished for making love while hunting or fishing on their wedding day.
Huh?

Essential Acid

About 80 percent of Americans don't eat enough essential fatty acids ("essential" to your diet because your body cannot make them) resulting in a number of problems from infertility to cardiovascular disease.

Every cell needs essential fatty acids, which are used to synthesize prostaglandins, hormone-like substances that were first discovered in the prostate gland. For starters, a prostaglandin (called E1) is needed to achieve an erection.

If you want to operate at peak sexual efficiency, make EFAs, especially omega-3s, part of your dietary arsenal. Seafood, especially fattier fish such as salmon, anchovies, sardines, bluefin tuna, and mackerel, are high in omega-3 fatty acids. Omega-3s can also help alleviate menstrual cramps, give you a glowing complexion, sharpen your brain, alleviate joint and muscle pain, and reduce depression, all of which help improve sexual vitality.

Eating fish and other foods high in omega-3s may also help protect the prostate gland. A thirty-year study published in the British journal *The Lancet* found that Swedish men who never or seldom ate fish were two to three times as likely to develop prostate cancer as men who ate moderate to high amounts of fish.

Enhances your sex drive: Some types of seafood, particularly oysters, mussels, and shark cartilage, are rich in natural substances called mucopolysaccharides, which can increase libido, potency, and the production of semen.

Improves genital blood flow: The omega-3 fatty acids in seafood can help reduce cholesterol levels and increase beneficial relaxation in arteries and blood vessels, improving blood flow to your genitals and heart.

Keeps you potent: Seafood is an excellent source of easy-to-digest, high-quality, low-calorie protein. Fish is rich in many essential vitamins and minerals including zinc (which is needed by both men and women for peak sexual performance) and magnesium (which relaxes smooth muscles lining blood vessels, allowing increased blood flow to the penis) that are important to a healthy libido and a good sex life.

Quick, light, energy source: While a heavy meal weighs you down and diverts blood from the genitals to the stomach and intestines for digestion, light meals (like fish) go easy on your digestive tract, so that you can save the blood flow for the real dessert.

Fish Fanatics Flourish

Casanova liked fish more than meat. His companion Angnolo Torredano, a great lover himself who died at age ninety-two in the arms of his teenage mistress and gave old Cass a few sexual tips ("Never ask for their phone number. Make them offer it."), made a powerful paella and called seafood the "food of life that makes it possible for this cold, old body to still enjoy the heat of passion."

Aztec emperors sent servants running to the sea to haul back buckets of fish for them to enjoy with their concubines. While across the world . . .

In Italy . . . Ancient Romans made a love sauce from fermented fish innards, blood, and gills and herbs, and served snails (which were kept in pens and fed wine, honey, and flour) as an aphrodisiac and hangover remedy. Roman gourmet Apicius recommended tuna (also noted by Aristophanes for its ability to increase virility), red mullet, sea bream, and squid as love foods.

The wanton Roman emperor Elagabalus, who liked to cruise around town in a chariot drawn by naked ladies (we kid you not), frequently dined on erotic fish meals and kept a fishing fleet just to catch eels so he could eat their roe.

In France . . . The French have always had a hankering for all kinds of seafood, from snails (they eat 40,000 metric tons each year) to oysters. They are responsible for the ultimate aphrodisiacal stew, bouillabaisse, a famous seafood soup that, according to French writer Charles Monselet, will get "chilly beauties, not a few, to do whatever you wish." (Hmmm, does that mean Uma Thurman?)

Renowned French mistress Madame de Pompadour, lover of Louis XV, called seafood a "prelude d'amour" and served Lou sole stuffed with truffles and mushrooms, cooked in champagne. Madame P. was a big spokeswoman for seafood, as her real last name was Poisson, French for fish. Good thing she changed it or we'd have a hairstyle called "fish" instead of pompadour.

Louis XV's other mistress, Comtesse du Barry, revived Louis's libido with pastilles (small lozenge-like candies) made from ambergris (a substance secreted by sperm whales) dubbed "The Powder of Joy" and "The Tablets of Love," and liked her shrimp cooked in sauterne sauce. Her countryman and fellow foodie Brillat-Savarin observed that a fish diet "gave to certain religious orders a reputation like that of Hercules." And French writer and priest Rabelais called fish "the food of harlots" and blamed the humble herring and other seafood eaten at Lent for prompting lascivious acts.

In England . . . Across the channel the English fueled their libidos with eels. *The Lucayos Cook Book,* written in 1660, gives a potent aphrodisiacal eel recipe entitled "Ye Collar Eele Recipe" that calls for both lovers to "take yor eeles and rub them with salt till all the skinne be quite taken off." What you do with your eels once the skin is off we can only guess, but would rather not. Perhaps this is the origin of the Brits' famous (and in our opinion, questionable) devotion to eel or green pie, which is made from jellied eel and chunks of fresh eel seasoned with Worcestershire sauce and vinegar.

....

naked supper

The seventeenth-century French restaurant Very's served seafood on a fish platter, in the middle of which lay a nude woman. (Why can't we get garnishes like *that* here in the States?) And in nineteenth-century Paris, upscale restaurants fed fish dishes to lovers who dined together in special "boudoir suites."

Prior to the French Revolution the upper crust enjoyed a wide variety of nude entertainment. People packed the Palais Royale Theatre to see a live stage play consisting of two actors having sex. Across town you could attend a naked supper at Madame Dervieux's brothel (brothels were frequented the way bars are today), or visit a restaurant (which was conveniently also a whorehouse) where naked men and women did a dance called "The Tums," which was supposed to help people digest dinner. Even the tableware was stimulating: Wineglass stems were often shaped like penises and bowls were decorated like the Greek and Roman vases of antiquity with depictions of orgies.

....

In Asia . . .

- Japanese aquatic aphrodisiacs include fugu (also called blowfish, it contains tetrodotoxin, a poison so potent the U.S. Food and Drug Administration says it can "produce rapid and violent death" if not properly prepared), sea urchin, and many varieties of sushi.
- In China, where the aphrodisiacal and nutritional value of seafood has been recognized for more than four thousand years, lovers go all night long by dining on scallops, shrimp, snails, lobster, steamed turtle soup, sautéed fish entrails, and a sauce called Nuoc-Man made from an extract of rotting fish. (Sounds like the Chinese took some culinary lessons from the Brits on this one.)

•Shark's fin soup, called yerchee, is also a popular Oriental love potion. The rich soup was a delicacy reserved for royalty and today it is popular at wedding feasts. After catching your shark you must cut off its fins and boil the meat for several days until it is white and tender. At $25 per pound, shark's fins are one of the most expensive fish dishes around. (And if people keep killing sharks for their fins, soon they won't be around at all.)

ALL the LittLe Fishes

Hundreds of seafood varieties are edible and many are powerful aphrodisiacs. Here's a few fish (and other sea creatures) you may wish to throw in your lover's dish.

Pompano: Described by Mark Twain as "delicious as the less conventional forms of sin." A small American fish, it weighs between 1 and 2 pounds, has a sweet, rich flavor, and can be grilled, sautéed, broiled, or baked whole.

Sea horse: We think this fish is better seen in an aquarium than served on a plate. In Asia, Chinese herbalists have prescribed sea horse powder for thousands of years, and about 20 million dried sea horses (they retail for as much as $500 per pound) are sold annually as an aphrodisiac and traditional Chinese remedy.

Sea horses have an elaborate mating ritual that takes three days and involves changing color, swimming up and down, and chasing each other around an aquatic maypole. At the end of the lengthy courtship the female deposits her eggs in the male's pouch. After several weeks of incubation and a difficult labor, sea horse super-dads give birth. Some species of sea horse are even monogamous, bonding for life and reinforcing the relationship by performing a mini courtship ritual every morning. Bonded males also tend to give birth to more babies, either by expanding the capacity of their pouch or increasing the production of the hormone prolactin.

(continued)

Starfish: Another popular aphrodisiac that we have yet to develop a taste for.

Octopus: This eight-armed guy has quite the reputation as an aphrodisiac, particularly among the Japanese, and is a popular culinary treat in Greece and other Mediterranean countries. In the U.S. he's called devil-fish because his rubbery flesh must be tenderized before cooking. Octopus meat is sweet and firm and can be fried, braised, baked, or sautéed.

Seaweed: In Jamaica folks consider a seaweed extract called Irish Moss (often mixed with milk, nutmeg, or rum) to be an aphrodisiac. Seaweed is high in potassium and iodine, which can help boost your sex life by nourishing the thyroid gland. (Thyroid problems can cause hormone imbalance and a low sex drive.) Many varieties of seaweed such as arame, nori, dulse, and wakame are tasty and highly nutritious.

Whether you like it or not, you've probably eaten seaweed in the form of a popular food additive called caragean, commonly used to make ice creams, salad dressings, and processed cheeses.

Sea Urchins: Sure, she resembles a hedgehog, and there's little meat to eat beneath that shell, but open her up and you'll discover five rose-colored ovaries that are considered an aphrodisiacal delicacy.

Apuleius, the second-century poet, philosopher, and rhetorician, made a love potion from sea urchins, cuttle-fish, spiced oysters, and lobsters.

Sea Slug: Known by Naples fishermen as sea Priapus (Priapus was the son of Dionysus and Aphrodite and a powerful phallic fertility deity who is always depicted with a gigantic hard-on) and as sea cucumbers, these aphrodisiacal mollusks are also hermaphrodites and swell and grow just like a penis when they are touched. The sea cucumber has a rubbery texture and is usually sold dehydrated in Asian markets.

Whale: Whale meat was so prized as a sexual stimulant in the Middle Ages that it was reserved for nobility. French kings were particularly fond of whale tongue. Eskimos considered mutak (whale) skin an aphrodisiac.

Bird's Nest Soup: This spicy soup is made from the edible nest of a bird called the swiftlet, which lives on about 140 islands in Southeast Asia. The edible nests, which are extremely dangerous to collect due to their remote locations in caves or on hazardous cliffs, are made from seaweed and fish spawn glued together by bird saliva. The brew is so highly revered in China for its ability to increase sex drive, reverse aging, and improve the complexion that nest smuggling is a multibillion-dollar business that is endangering the swiftlets. A kilogram of bird's nest can sell for as much as $4,500 and a bowl in a good Hong Kong restaurant can cost as much as $60.

Crayfish: Popular New Orleans chow (head and all), these crustaceans (also called crawfish, crawdads, écrevisses, and yabbies), are closely related to lobster and are highly regarded as a love food in the Mediterranean, where they are boiled in oil with salt, pepper, garlic, and other spices. Cook them like lobster (until they turn bright red), eat them with your hands, and enjoy sucking the sweet, succulent meat out of the small shells.

Conch: If oysters aren't native to your waters your next best bet is *Strombus gigas,* the queen conch. Caribbean natives swear they are an aphrodisiac and a source of virility, particularly the tail end, which is bitten off and eaten while the conch is still squirming. "Hey, mon, conch put de lead in ya pencil." Like other aphrodisiacal fish, the conch is very fertile, laying half a million eggs at a time. Maybe conch, which is the national dish of the Bahamas and is incorporated in everything from chowder to cerviche, is the real reason the Caribbean is the place for honeymooners. Look for the snail-like creatures in Caribbean markets and, unless you like rubber hot dogs, make sure to tenderize the meat in a little lime juice before cooking.

Aphrodite's crown jewels: caviar, Lobster, salmon, and shrimp

caviar: Aphrodite's Platinum card

Caviar is to dining what a sable coat is to a girl in evening dress.

—Ludwiq Bemelmans, author of *Madeline*

Caviar is the platinum standard of aphrodisiacs—expensive, exquisite, glamorous, and bursting with nutrients that enhance sexual vitality. Caviar slips across your palate like a perfect night of lovemaking, evaporating in the morning mist like a dream, leaving a delicious memory on the tip of your tongue.

Enjoyed by czars and czarinas, kings, princes, queens, and emperors (as well as a couple of Cossacks), caviar, like other extravagant aphrodisiacs, fois gras, and truffles, symbolizes decadence, and its elusiveness alone makes it a potent aphrodisiac.

Great caviar is like great sex. The more you eat the more you want, and at up to $125 an ounce for the real stuff, it will shred

catherine II and caviar

When childless Catherine II of Russia was having trouble producing an heir for the empire with her husband, the grandson of Peter the Great, she turned to caviar. She ordered her chef to cook a caviar-drenched dinner that included a fine sturgeon, which she shared not with her husband but with Saltikoff, an officer of the guard. Lo and behold the caviar worked (as did Saltikoff), and nine months later she gave birth to an heir.

Lucky for Catherine (and Salty) there was no such thing as DNA testing back then.

your wallet faster than a bad-girl blonde in Vegas. Thank God that just a dab will do ya.

The Romans were so fond of caviar that they had servants carry live sturgeon in buckets all the way from the Caspian Sea to Rome.

The Greeks started their version of a cocktail party (otherwise known as an orgy) by passing around hors d'oeuvres that consisted of caviar, oysters, and roasted grasshoppers.

Alexander the Great, who learned how to produce caviar from Darius, the king of Persia, introduced the succulent sturgeon eggs to the West. The Persians praised caviar as a great love food, and caviar was frequently served in French sex salons.

As an incentive to complete *Crime and Punishment,* Dostoyevsky's wife fed him caviar each time he finished a chapter. No wonder it's over forty chapters long!

Caviar contains dozens of nutrients that are good for your sexual vitality, including the amino acid arginine, which increases the body's level of nitric oxide, a key ingredient in the erection equation. So ladies, let him have the last spoonful; it will pay off in the bedroom.

If you have rock star cash you may want to spoon-feed him an appetizer called "Harlot's Eggs," made by combining pimento with anchovy paste, chopped chives, a squeeze of lemon, and half a cup of caviar.

Labels Matter

Caviar is the edible, salted eggs, or "roe," of several species of fish. Real caviar comes only from sturgeon, an ancient (250 million years, to be precise), toothless, endangered fish that lives in the sea and spawns in fresh water.

Other fish eggs can be sold as caviar, but the label must identify the name of the fish, for example "salmon caviar" or "whitefish caviar." In the United States, labeling regulations insist that if the label says only "caviar" then it must be from a sturgeon.

The Incredible Erotic Egg

All types of eggs, including fish eggs, are symbols of fertility, and are used to stimulate sexual desire. The yolk, particularly when eaten raw, is considered the most sexually potent part of the egg. A Jewish folk remedy for sterility calls for eating an egg with a double yolk. Here are a few other ways to reach eggstacy.

From France: Drop a raw egg yolk into a glass of cognac and enjoy at breakfast. (No wonder these guys can't win a war.)

From Casanova: "You shall feel all through the night the ardor of my devotions. . . . I have taken nothing today but a cup of chocolate and a salad of eggs dressed with oil from Lucca and Marseilles vinegar. . . . I shall be all right when I have distilled the whites of the eggs, one by one, into your amorous soul."

From the Middle East: According to *The Perfumed Garden,* a manual of Arabian erotic techniques: "He who boils asparagus and then fries them in fat, and then pours upon them the yolks of eggs with pounded condiments, and eats every day of this dish, will grow very strong for the coitus, and find in it a stimulant for his amorous desires."

Another popular Arabic love brunch is fried eggs drenched with honey and served with toast.

From Down Under: The Australian Aborigines make an aphrodisiac potion from powdered aged emu eggshell that is used by both men and women.

From the Islands: In the Philippines sea turtle eggs are gathered and sold as an aphrodisiac.

From India: To prevent impotence, eat a half-boiled egg mixed with ginger juice and honey every night for a month.

HeaLth food, russian styLe

Russians have regarded caviar as a health food for centuries and used it to prevent rickets, decrease recovery time following surgery, and as a hangover remedy.

The satiny eggs are low in calories (about 40 per tablespoon), light, easy to digest, protein rich, and high in omega-3 fatty acids. They contain acetylcholine, a neurotransmitter important to memory and general mental function, which may increase the body's ability to tolerate alcohol. A big plus since caviar is best enjoyed with chilled vodka or champagne. Nostrovia!

Before being sold as caviar sturgeon roe is separated from the membranes encasing the eggs, washed, rubbed with salt to preserve and cure them, and then packaged. There are three kinds of "real" caviar: beluga, osetra, and sevruga.

Beluga is the largest grained and the most prized. Beluga hails from the biggest sturgeon, reaching 20 feet and weighing up to 1,800 pounds. The female doesn't start laying the delicately flavored gray eggs until she is 18 to 20 years old.

Beluga was Pablo Picasso's favorite caviar. To pay for his caviar stash he would send money wrapped in a signed sketch. Inevitably, the sketch was worth more than the cash . . . and the caviar.

The most costly caviar in the world is Almas (Russian for "diamond"). This white beluga caviar comes from fish that are more than a century old. (In general, older fish produce the best caviar.) The rare eggs are packaged in 24K solid gold tins and cost more than $23,000 for 35 ounces.

If you can afford this you've got too much money! How about skipping the Almas and donating some to a worthy cause?

Osetra, the fabled "golden caviar," is golden amber to brown in color, and has a medium grain and a sweet almond-like flavor. The osetra sturgeon matures between the ages of 12 and 15 years and are smaller than the beluga, weighing between 100 and 300 pounds.

Ian Fleming, the James Bond creator, favored this caviar.

Sevruga has a creamy texture and a stronger flavor than beluga or osetra. The female starts to lay her small gray eggs when she is between 5 and 7 years old. Sevruga is the best value of imported caviars and travels well.

The famous French leader Charles de Gaulle was a Sevruga fan.

Low supply and high demand make caviar pricey. The number of sturgeon continues to decline, and unless measures are taken to increase the population, these fish may soon become extinct.

Sturgeon wasn't always an endangered species. During the 1800s sturgeon were abundant in California, the Pacific Northwest, and on the East Coast (in New York and New Jersey caviar was so plentiful that it was called "Albany Beef") and America had a thriving caviar business. The salty eggs were widely exported to Europe (where they were sometimes labeled as "Russian imported caviar" and shipped back to the States) and served for free in bars to enhance thirst and beer sales. However, by the middle of the twentieth century overfishing and pollution destroyed the domestic American sturgeon to the point of extinction. Today, only imported caviar is available in America.

Good caviar is balanced. It should have a nice sheen and taste of the sea without being too salty or oily. A bit chewy, the eggs should have a slight crunch and pop in your mouth.

The best way to enjoy caviar is to open the chilled tin (caviar should be kept between 32° F and 45° F to prevent deterioration) right before eating. Feed your lover directly from the tin with a nonmetallic spoon. Silver and stainless steel can give caviar a

other Roes to Hoe

Fortunately for the environmentally conscious caviar connoisseur with bills to pay, there are other domestic and imported roes to enjoy that are delicious and have the same aphrodisiacal qualities as the real McCoy.

Fresh American Paddlefish caviar comes from fish that spawn in rivers in Tennessee, Alabama, and Missouri. The caviar is pearl-gray, has a firm texture, and is similar in taste to Sevruga caviar.

Bowfin (Amia calva) or "Choupique Caviar" comes from an ancient, boney fish that swims in Louisiana's bayous. The eggs are black and firm and have a bright, distinctive flavor.

Freshwater Salmon caviar is very popular on the sushi circuit in Japan where it is called ikura and comes from farm-raised chinook and coho salmon. The large, bright orange, juicy roe has an intense salmon flavor and pops when you bite it.

Hackeback caviar comes from both shovel nose sturgeon that live wild in the Mississippi river system, and farmed white sturgeon in California. The roe is black and has a sweet, nutty flavor.

Lumpfish caviar is imported from Canada, Iceland, and Scandinavia. The small, chewy eggs are black or bright red and have a slightly fishy taste.

metallic taste. If your gold spoon is in the dishwasher, just use a plastic one.

Serve in the bedroom (our favorite caviar cave) accompanied by plenty of champagne or ice-cold vodka. (Put the vodka bottle directly in your freezer and leave it there. It won't freeze; its alcohol content is too high.)

Caviar can also be served on thin pieces of buttered toast or on little buckwheat pancakes called blini with a touch of sour cream.

For a double aphro pop, try topping raw oysters with a touch of caviar.

{ BLini: caviar's surfboard }

1 package active dry yeast
¼ cup warm water, about 85° F
1 tablespoon sugar
2 cups flour
2 cups milk
1 teaspoon salt
3 eggs, separated
1 tablespoon butter, melted

1. In a small bowl combine yeast, warm water, and sugar. Stir mixture well, cover the bowl with a clean dish towel, and set in a warm place until yeast starts to foam, about 10 minutes.
2. In a separate bowl, whisk together flour, milk, salt, egg yolks, and melted butter. Stir in yeast mixture. Cover bowl with a clean dish towel and let batter rise in a warm place until almost double in bulk, about 1½ hours.
3. Beat egg whites until soft peaks form and fold into batter.
4. Heat a 10-inch greased griddle or skillet until a drop of cold water sizzles and sputters when dropped onto pan surface. Make a few thin pancakes at a time by pouring batter from a spoon onto hot griddle or skillet. Cook until light-brown, flipping once. Stack cooked pancakes on paper towels.

Top each blini with a little caviar (about ½ teaspoon) and a dab of sour cream. Alternative toppings include sautéed mushrooms, or fresh sliced fruit or berries mixed with sweetened ricotta, or marscapone cheese.

Makes 24 two-inch cakes

LOBSTERS, SEXUAL DYNAMOS FROM THE SEA

I was in the Virgin Islands once. I met a girl. We ate lobster and drank piña coladas. At sunset we made love like sea otters. That was a pretty good day.

—BILL MURRAY in *GROUNDHOG DAY*

When it comes to the foods of love, *Homarus americanus,* the American lobster, is unique. Once so abundant that the Pilgrims considered him poor man's meat and Maine fishermen used him as bait, today lobsters are a lusciously lascivious luxury item. The sensual pleasure of devouring a whole lobster is in itself an aphrodisiac, a ritual we reserve for celebrating anniversaries.

Start by popping a pair of lobsters into the pot. Ten to fifteen minutes later, pull the steaming, bright red crustaceans from the simmering water. Ripping the shells apart with your bare hands (after they cool), you free the moist flesh, dip the succulent meat in melted butter, and enter an aquatic wonderland of rich sweetness. Add a touch of liquid gold with a wonderful sauterne, chardonnay, or champagne and serve with an ear of corn, a wedge of brie, and a baguette and you are in for a lust fest, memories of which will stick with you when the ground is covered with snow and summer fun is a distant memory.

Cooking a live lobster and devouring it whole is a primal event and an all-or-nothing experience. We recommend that you dive in with abandon, forgoing the bib (there's nothing sexy about a bib unless it's the only thing you're wearing) and foraging for every morsel of tender meat with any tools that are at your disposal—nutcrackers, sledgehammers, bare hands, teeth. Like hot sex, devouring a lobster is erotic and messy. That's what makes it such fun. For a lubricant we recommend plenty of melted butter. Here's the systematic way to proceed.

1. Start with the claws. Tear them off, crack them open, and pull out and eat the meat.

2. Next, move on to the tail. Being careful not to splash each other with lobster juice (or not), use a twisting motion to separate the tail from the body. Pull the meat out from the thicker end with your fingers and eat.

3. Now it's time to attack the trunk. Separate the back of the lobster shell from the body and eat any bits of meat adjacent to the walking leg joints. Whether or not to eat the lobster liver, called the tomalley (the soft green stuff), is a matter of personal choice. Some people consider tomalley a delicacy. Others think eating it is disgusting. The Cooking Couple split right down the middle on this one: Ellen yea, Michael nay.

4. Still hungry? There's a bit of meat inside each of the six walking legs, which can be obtained either by pressing on the legs with your thumb and index finger or sucking the meat out like a straw.

5. Forget the moist towelettes. Remember, cleaning up means showering together.

Don't take our word for it. For a graphic rendition of the seductive art of lobster-eating, rent *Tom Jones* and watch Mrs. Waters and Tom suck lobster meat from the shell and make a hasty exit to the bedroom to feed their sexual appetites. For a more modern lobster tale, rent *Flashdance* and watch Jennifer Beals seduce her dinner companion with lobster meat and hot feet. Or you could choose the Oscar-winning *Annie Hall* and watch Woody Allen and Diane Keaton, a pair of New York apartment dwellers, conduct a lobster hunt in their bathroom. Although not erotic (in some locales Woody Allen is used as a contraceptive), it shows the lengths that New Yorkers will go to for a lobster dinner.

Hey Baby, Wanna Dance?

Quick on his feet (after all, he does have sixteen of them), the male lobster literally serenades his intended with a Salomelike erotic dance of desire to win her affections. No dance, no nookie! "You put your right claw in, you take your right claw out. You put your left claw in and you shake it all about. You do the lobster pokey and you turn yourself around. That's what it's all about!"

The lobster lambada starts when the female is ready to molt (sort of like changing into "something a little more comfortable"). Then, to attract a mate, she releases a sex perfume called a pheromone, contained in her urine, near her chosen lover's den. Male lobsters can detect pheromones in the water using chemoreceptors located on their antennae. In lobster society the females do the choosing, generally selecting the largest male in the vicinity.

Not only do these pheromones attract prospective males, they also reduce aggressiveness so that the female doesn't become lunch. (This isn't a cunnilingus joke. Lobsters are scavengers and known to eat just about anything, including each other.) The male lobster responds by moving the pheromone-saturated water with his swimmerets (Who names these things?) into his apartment so that her perfume permeates it. He then comes out of his den, claws raised aggressively, ready to tango. She curbs his angry advance by either turning away or engaging in a brief boxing match.

Now the real fun begins, when the male and female strike up the band and do the Rock Lobster. In an elaborate sexual waltz, the female strokes the male with her antennae and they serenade each other by clicking their claws. (*Boléro* by Ravel seems to be #1 on the current lobster hit parade.) After about fifteen minutes of musical foreplay the female places her claws on the male's head to let him know that she is ready to mate. The pair then retire to his crib for several days of cohabitation and the occasional boxing match. (Scientists theorize that the male may jab the female to determine how soon she will shed her shell so they can do it.)

Lobsters make love in the missionary position, belly to belly, which is rare in the animal kingdom. After the female has lost her shell, the male carefully turns his lover over with his legs, enters her with a rigid pair of swimmerets, and ejaculates into a seminal receptacle that sits between the female's fourth and fifth pair of legs. This whole process takes about 8 seconds.

As with many other species, at this point the male lights a cigarette, mentions something about calling soon, and scuttles off to the nearest clam shack, leaving the female to carry on for the next twenty months or so on her own. ("What's the matter with me, Sheila? I fall for that stupid dance *every* time!" "Honey, I gotta tell you the truth. You gotta stop thinking with your ovaries. You know men only want to get between your fourth and fifth set of legs. You want love, you get yourself a nice rich crab or monkfish. They treat you right.")

After recovering from sex the female leaves the male's den and takes up residence elsewhere until her shell hardens. Then she lays her eggs, passing them over the seminal receptacle where the sperm has been stored. Next, she carries the fertilized eggs glued to her abdomen by a sticky substance. After releasing thousands of eggs, the female simply swims away looking for her next dance, without a care in the world for what happens to her tiny, helpless brood.

The life of a lobster is tough. Only a tiny percentage of lobsterlings survive to become large enough to feed human lust. (Many creatures, including seals, raccoon, cod, eels, and flounder, love to sup on them.) Lobsters molt seven times in the first year and it takes them five to seven years just to reach a pound in weight. Fortunately for us and them, lobsters have a few tricks up their sleeves (actually eight sleeves, to be precise)—they lay many eggs, are protected by strong armor, have lethal claws that can literally break a finger, and can regenerate parts of themselves that are torn or bitten off. If they can escape all the perils of lobster life, they can reach a ripe old age of sixty or seventy and fatten up to as much as forty pounds.

Hey, but maybe this is more information on the lovable lobster than you want. And we know it's more information than you need. So let's get on to the good stuff, like how to enjoy these amorous crustaceans.

lobster trivia

- A female lobster is called a hen. A male lobster is called a cock.
- A lobster that weighs about one pound is called a chicken.
- A lobster without claws is called a pistol.
- *Berries* are lobster eggs, and *bug* is slang for lobster.
- The first chamber of a lobster trap is called the kitchen.
- When a lobsterman has "shorts on" it means he has caught lobsters that are smaller than the legal size.
- The first pair of swimmerets under the tail are hard on males and soft on females. Females also have a wider tail and a small rectangular-shaped sperm receptacle between their walking legs.
- Today lobstermen band lobsters' claws to keep them from eating each other. (Lobsters are cannibals, which is why they are not farmed like other seafood.) They used to peg the claws, but this led to infection.
- Lobsters continue to grow throughout their life. The record for the world's largest lobster goes to a Nova Scotia specimen caught in 1977 that weighed 44 lbs., 6 oz., and was between three and four feet long.
- Lobsters have poor vision and smell through their feet. Their kidneys are in their head and their teeth are in their stomach. (What was God smoking when she made this animal?)
- Lobsters probably feel no pain because they lack a central nervous system and cerebral cortex, the part of the brain where painful stimuli is usually processed.

Seven Rules for a Lobster Love Affair

If a lobster didn't look like a sci-fi monster, people would be less able to drop him alive into boiling water.

–george carlin

Rule number 1. Buy them alive and lively. As with all seafood (and many other foods, for that matter) the better the raw material, the better the meal and aphrodisiacal effect. So look for lobsters that are alive and kicking.

Rule number 2. Buy hard-shell lobsters only. Lobsters molt frequently to make room for their growing bodies and may be in some stage of molting during the summer and early fall. When the ocean water starts to warm, lobsters form a new soft shell under their old armor.

During the molting process, lobsters dehydrate (which shrinks the meat) so that they can squeeze through a tiny opening in their old shell. They emerge with a new shell and shrunken meat, which is chewy and shriveled. Soft-shell lobsters taste waterlogged and are a real disappointment. The way to tell whether

---

"you're getting sleepy, sleepy, sleepy . . ."

Here's a great party trick that is sure to impress your dinner date. To hypnotize your beast, stand it on its head on a flat surface with claws placed in front and tail curling inward. Rub up and down its shell with your hand, especially between the eyes. Do it well and your yogi lobster may remain in the headstand position all by itself.

Although this does put them to sleep, lobsters usually wake up as soon as they realize they are about to be boiled alive.

your lobster will be mushy or succulent is to look at the claws. Lobsters that have not yet molted have black mottling on the underside of their claws.

Rule number 3. Decide ahead of time who does the dirty work. In our household, Ellen dumps the lobsters into the water and Michael comforts her when she runs out of the kitchen screaming. ("Ellen, I told you not to name them.")

Rule number 4. Never name your lobsters.

Rule number 5. To keep them alive and kicking, store the lobsters in a loosely closed brown paper bag (lobsters need to breathe) in the refrigerator until cooking time.

Rule number 6. K.I.S.S. Keep it simple, sweetheart. No, we don't mean the rock band in clown makeup, although the shoes are nice. We mean that starting with good quality ingredients and cooking them in a simple, straightforward, easy way is usually best. Our favorite way to cook lobsters is in a large pot of boiling water. Plunge the lobsters into the water head first. When the water comes back to a boil, start your timer. The average 1¼ pound lobster takes about 12 minutes to cook after the water starts to boil again. Check our Aphrodite Menu for Amour (page 107) for other preparation and cooking methods.

Rule number 7. Skip the silly-looking bib unless you're wearing a rented tux or eating in the nude.

The Mighty Salmon

Old impotent Alden from Waldern
Ate salmon to heat him to scaldin'
'twas just the ticket
to stiffen his wicket
This salmon of amorous Alden.

—Anonymous

Wild salmon, the toughest and bravest fish in the sea, imparts virility to anyone who eats it. Dubbed "The King of Fish," the colorful, regal, tasty salmon is the most heroic and aphrodisiacal fish, swimming thousands of miles against terrible odds just to mate. Sex therapist Dr. Ruth Westheimer has called salmon "the new aphrodisiac," and according to Ayurvedic medicine salmon is a strengthening food and sexual stimulant.

A fabulous, versatile food that's rich in many nutrients that fuel sexual vitality from omega-3 fatty acids to high-quality protein, salmon should get a starring role on every lover's plate. Salmon is like that perfect little black dress. Whether you grill, poach, or broil it, accessorize lightly with a touch of butter and aphrodisiacal herbs, or go for a more assertive sauce. Whatever the occasion, salmon is always light and right, a perfect foundation for an aphrodisiacal night.

Salmon was the most prized fish in ancient Ireland, where it was roasted and served with honey. In the famous tale from the *Fenian Cycle of Irish Mythology* there is a magical salmon, called the "Salmon of Knowledge," who lived in the River Boyne and ate hazelnuts. According to the legend, the first person to eat the magical salmon would have knowledge of all things. A young Celtic poet (at the time, poets were the equivalent of today's rock stars) named Demne tasted the salmon after his teacher caught it and received three gifts: magic, great insight, and the power of

on the seventh day he partied

Six days a week Saint Finian, an Irish monk and follower of Saint Patrick, lived on bread and water. On Sundays he dined on two aphrodisiacs, salmon and mead.

Mead (honey wine) and salmon have been major players on the Irish wedding circuit, fueling first-night bliss at least since the fifth century. Salmon for strength, mead for . . . lubrication. Irish monks first produced mead as a medicine, and quickly realized that the potent brew made people, whether sick or healthy, feel great fast.

While today couples receive a champagne toast, in medieval times mead was the essential wedding night lubricant. Drinking the strong, delectable beverage was believed to be the best way to start a marriage and a family (as well as have a good time) because it was believed to enhance fertility and virility. The groom, plied with plenty of mead, was frequently carried to the bridal bed by his buddies. If a baby popped out nine months later, mead got the credit.

As a wedding gift the bride and groom received enough mead for the next lunar month, which is where the term *honeymoon* comes from.

words. Demne changed his name to Dylan and, well, you know the rest of the story.

Like oysters, salmon lead a double life. While oysters are androgynous, salmon are anadromous, which means they live in the sea and then adapt to fresh water. Their entire life cycle is dedicated to spawning. After spending one to four years at sea, these mighty fish travel hundreds and sometimes thousands of miles to their place of birth, freshwater rivers that flow into the sea. They fight their way upstream by hurling their iridescent bodies against the rapidly flowing waters. Many die in this effort to deposit and fertilize eggs in one specific spot. Once their mission is accomplished, Pacific salmon die, while Atlantic salmon live to spawn again.

Most wild salmon come from the northern waters of the Pacific; the Alaska coast being a prime source. Most farm-raised salmon are native to the Atlantic waters off the east coast of the United States and Europe, though today salmon is farmed throughout the world. Salmon farming accounts for more than half of the salmon that is eaten today.

While farm-raised salmon tends to be cheap and plentiful compared to their wild brothers and sisters, as an aphrodisiac it pales in comparison. (Farm-raised salmon are white and are fed pigment to turn them shades of red.) Wild salmon is more flavorful and has a firmer, meatier texture. Unlike wild salmon, the farmed fish never have to fight their way upstream to spawn. Wild salmon are oiler and richer in omega-3s than farmed salmon due to thousands of years of natural selection, providing them with the fat reserves necessary for migration and spawning.

There are five varieties of wild Pacific salmon:

·King (also called Chinook): The best of the bunch. They average twenty pounds, have pink to red flesh, are high in healthy omega-3 fats, and have a wonderfully rich flavor.

·Red Sockeye (also called red or blueback): *Sockeye* is an Indian word meaning "best of fishes," literally "fish of fishes" in Salish. These salmon are moist and flavorful, high in fat, and have a distinctive, deep-red color. The male has a hooked lower jaw and both male and female have a slightly humped back. Sockeye has a complex, earthy flavor that is intensified by grilling or smoking.

·Silver (also called coho): This species averages eight to twelve pounds, has orange-red flesh, a milder, more delicate flavor due to the lower oil content, and a finer texture than king or sockeye.

·Chum: These average about nine pounds. The flavor is delicate and the fat content is lower than king and sockeye. They are also called "dog" salmon because the males grow enlarged canine teeth at spawning time. Perhaps vampire salmon would be a better description.

Aphro sauces for Aphro salmon

Here are some quick and easy ways to spike salmon with aphrodisiacs.

•*Pesto:* Brush salmon fillets or steaks with pesto. Top with herbed bread crumbs and bake or broil.

•*Rosemary Red Onion:* Place salmon fillets or steaks on a bed of rosemary and sliced red onion. Top with additional rosemary and sliced red onion and roast or bake.

•*Zucchini Butter Sauce:* Chop ¾ pound medium zucchini and simmer in water covered for 15 minutes. Purée cooked zucchini with 1 tablespoon butter and salt and pepper to taste, until smooth. Serve over warm, poached salmon. For a spicier version add 1 teaspoon of curry powder to the sauce.

•*Honey Mustard Sauce:* Mix ¼ cup Dijon mustard with 2 tablespoons honey, 1 tablespoon vegetable oil, and 1 tablespoon cider vinegar. Use as a basting sauce for grilled or broiled salmon.

•*Herb Sauce:* Mix ½ cup sour cream or yogurt with ¼ cup mayonnaise, 3 tablespoons minced fresh aphrodisiacal herbs, 1 tablespoon vinegar, and salt and pepper to taste. Use as a sauce for grilled, poached, or broiled salmon.

•*Chili Avocado Sauce:* Purée one medium ripe avocado with ½ cup sour cream or yogurt, 1 teaspoon chili powder, ½ teaspoon cumin, 1 teaspoon lime juice, and salt, pepper, and hot sauce to taste. Serve as a sauce for grilled, baked, sautéed, or roasted salmon.

•*Teriyaki:* Mix ¼ cup soy sauce with 2 tablespoons honey, 1 tablespoon rice vinegar, ½ teaspoon grated ginger, 1 clove chopped garlic, 1 teaspoon toasted sesame oil, and red chile pepper flakes to taste. Marinade salmon for 1 to 2 hours before grilling, broiling, baking, or roasting.

•Pink: This is the smallest type of Pacific salmon, weighing in at only two to three pounds, and is the most plentiful. It has a light rose-colored flesh and a subtle flavor.

America's favorite supper fish (more tuna is eaten, but most of it is canned), salmon is available whole or cut into steaks and boneless fillets, and comes fresh, canned, and frozen. Salmon is a joy to prepare and lends itself to a wide variety of cooking methods. Because salmon has a firm texture and high fat content it doesn't dry out easily or fall apart, making it a great grilling fish.

Native American Indians living in the Pacific Northwest, who celebrated the appearance of the first salmon of the year with great ceremony, would split the salmon open, thread it on a stick (the way kids roast marshmallows today), and place it at an angle in front of an open fire. With modern grills and barbecues it's a lot easier to make great grilled salmon now, so give it a shot. You won't be disappointed. Just place a salmon steak on a hot, well-greased grill and baste with butter, oil, or a favorite marinade. Turn once, giving about four to six minutes per side, per inch.

Salmon also cures beautifully. The process of smoking salmon was developed in Russia in the eighteenth century, where it was popularized by many Jewish families who had a lust for lox. (The German word for salmon is *lachs,* and the Yiddish word is *laks.*) As Russian Jews immigrated to the United States (particularly New York, particularly, particularly Brooklyn) in the early twentieth century, they brought their lox with them.

Besides Brooklyn, many lesser countries famous for their smoked salmon include Scotland, Ireland, and Scandinavia, where the salmon is smoked and cured with dill, salt, sugar, and pepper and called Gravad Lax.

shrimp, Nature's Finger Food

Shrimp is the fruit of the sea. You can barbecue it, boil it, broil it, bake it, sauté it. Dey's, uh, shrimp-kabobs, shrimp creole, shrimp gumbo. Pan fried, deep fried, stir fried. There's pineapple shrimp, lemon shrimp, coconut shrimp, pepper shrimp, shrimp soup, shrimp stew, shrimp salad, shrimp and potatoes, shrimp burger, shrimp sandwich. That—that's about it.

–Bubba in *Forrest Gump*

Shrimp are nature's perfect finger food: firm enough to hold together and eat with the hands, yet fleshy, sweet, succulently light, and flavorful. The Romans knew what they were doing when they ate shrimp as a prelude to making love. Japanese lovers looking for a boost favor a dish called ebi odori—live shrimp that are shelled, gutted, split, and eaten on balls of rice while they are still wriggling.

In the Caribbean, some natives eat live shrimp while they make love, and in South America, seviche (raw shrimp and other shellfish marinated in lime juice), often spiked with chile peppers, is served on beds of ice as a potent aphrodisiac.

Captain James Cook's shipmate recorded one of the best aphrodisiacal fish tales on an exploratory voyage to the Pacific in the eighteenth century. According to the shipmate it was Pacific Island King Lapetamaka II's duty to deflower every maiden on the island. (Tough job, this king business.) Required to have sex eight to ten times a day, the King attributed his sexual vitality to a simple precoital dish of shrimp with spices and pineapple.

While the word *shrimp* comes from the English *shrimpe*, meaning "a small person" and the Swedish *skrumpa,* "to shrink," there's nothing skimpy about shrimp. The United States consumes more shrimp than any other country, about 850 million pounds annually. The United States imports about half of the world's production, mostly from Thailand, Ecuador, Indonesia,

The skinny on shrimp

Shrimp, like other crustaceans, are low in fat and calories. A three-ounce serving (about a dozen large, cooked shrimp) has only 90 calories and 1.5 grams of fat most of which is unsaturated. Shrimp are high in cholesterol. That three-ounce portion contains over a third of the recommended daily intake for cholesterol (300 milligrams), but recent scientific research is showing that for most people, saturated fat plays a bigger role in raising cholesterol levels than the amount of cholesterol eaten. If you are watching your cholesterol level, eat shrimp in moderation and avoid shrimp that are fried, sautéed in a lot of butter, or served with a fattening sauce.

China, and India. (Shrimp caught in the wild tend to be more flavorful and have a firmer texture.)

Shrimp live in every ocean and lend themselves to a wide variety of preparations and cuisines. You can sauté or broil them for a few minutes in butter or oil and a bit of garlic for a savory scampi, or use them in more complex aphrodisiacal dishes such as prawn vindaloo, Caribbean coconut shrimp, jambalaya, or gumbo. They're also great on the grill, and wonderful cooked and served cold as shrimp cocktail. Plus, shrimp cook very quickly and freeze well, so you can always have some on hand.

There are hundreds of varieties of shrimp, all of which fall into two categories, "warm" or "cold" water, and come in three colors: white, pink, and brown. White shrimp taste best. They have a delicate flavor and lack the iodine aftertaste that is common in the cheaper brown variety.

Most shrimp are flash frozen at sea and then sold in either a frozen or thawed state. Frozen shrimp, whether cooked or raw, should be defrosted in the refrigerator or placed in a Ziploc bag and immersed in a large bowl of cold water for thirty to forty-five minutes.

When buying raw, defrosted, shell-on shrimp, look for clean shrimp with spotless shells (spots indicate poor handling) that are securely attached. The meat should smell sweet (if you detect the odor of ammonia, the shrimp are past their prime) and be firm, not mushy. Shelled shrimp should be whole and look clean and bright.

Size matters. Shrimp are sold either by the number in a pound (31/35, for example, means 31 to 35 shrimp per pound) or by size designation—small, medium, large, and jumbo. While a certain recipe may call for a particular size of shrimp, feel free to vary the size based on availability, price, and your preferences. If medium shrimp are on sale and the recipe calls for large, go for the medium. Use the same weight of shrimp called for in the recipe, just cook the shrimp for a minute or two less when substituting

shrimp, weighing the options

With so many sizes and styles of shrimp on the market, substituting one type for another makes sense. We suggest buying ¾ pound of raw, unshelled shrimp per person, or ⅓ to ½ pound of shelled cooked shrimp per person. Here are the basic equivalents to keep in mind when shopping for shrimp.

1 pound of raw unpeeled shrimp = ¾ pound of raw peeled shrimp
1 pound of raw shrimp = ½ pound of cooked shrimp (Shrimp shrinks a lot when cooked.)

While the number of shrimp you get in each size category can vary between fish stores, here's a general guideline for raw, unpeeled shrimp.

Jumbo = 8 to 10 shrimp per pound
Large = 10 to 25 shrimp per pound
Medium = 26 to 40 shrimp per pound
Small = 41 to 60 shrimp per pound

smaller shrimp and a minute or two longer when substituting larger shrimp.

The biggest mistake people make when preparing shrimp is overcooking. Regardless of the preparation method, shrimp cook in just a few minutes, and are done when the shell becomes pink or coral and the flesh turns from translucent to opaque. Larger shrimp take slightly longer to cook, so adjust your recipe accordingly. Start timing as soon as you toss the shrimp in the pot, and remember to check them frequently.

Shrimp Prep: Naked or Dressed?

You can cook shrimp with or without the shells. Shelled shrimp absorb more flavor from the dish you are creating, but the shells themselves add flavor to the sauce, and leaving them on saves time. We recommend leaving the shells on for grilling (unless shrimp are marinated) to prevent the shrimp from drying out. We generally take the shells off for dishes where the shrimp are hidden in a sauce or combined with other ingredients in soups, stews, and seafood dishes like paella, bouillabaisse, gumbo, and jambalaya.

"Devein, Devein . . ."

To devein or not to devein, that is the question. We generally leave the veins on for smaller shrimp. (You have better things to do than stand at the sink all day ripping out tiny shrimp veins.) Plus, small shrimp end up looking pretty ratty when you mess with them too much.

We tend to remove veins from larger shrimp, especially when the veins are black and visible. To devein larger shrimp, simply make a slit along the back with a paring knife and lift out the vein. You can avoid the whole deveining dilemma by simply buying easy-to-peel shrimp, which come with the shell split and the vein removed.

Fish: it's an aphrodisiac snap

Seafood is extremely easy to prepare, which is why it is one of our favorite love foods. Occasionally it's fun to make a dish that's a bit more challenging, but most of the time our amour menu motto is K.I.S.S. (Keep it simple, sweetheart). You don't want to spend the whole evening cooking.

While you can find plenty of complicated seafood recipes concocted by sadomasochistic celebrity chefs (Anyone for smoked salmon Napoleon with osetra caviar and wasabi crème fraîche?) that take even an experienced cook half a day to prepare, we recommend buying the freshest fish you can and enhancing its flavor with herbs and spices, a touch of butter or lemon juice, and a kiss.

When fish is fresh there is no need for complicated sauces and extravagant accompaniments. Remember, when it comes to fish, Aphrodite has already done the work for you.

The cooking couple's aphrodite menu for amour

{ pistachio-basil salmon }

The combination of basil, pistachios, and garlic (all of which are aphrodisiacs) works beautifully with salmon. The pistachio-basil butter can be made in advance and kept in the refrigerator for several days.

¼ cup fresh basil leaves

¼ cup pistachios

1 garlic clove

¼ cup butter

1 teaspoon lemon juice

Salt and freshly ground black pepper to taste

2 salmon fillets or steaks (about 8 ounces each)

Lemon wedges for garnish

1. Preheat oven to 375° F.

2. Place pistachios, basil, and garlic in a food processor or blender and process until finely chopped. Add butter, lemon juice, salt, and pepper and process into a smooth paste. Spread 2 to 3 table-spoons of pistachio butter on each piece of salmon. (You can refrigerate leftovers for several days and use as a spread or toss with pasta.)

3. Bake salmon in preheated oven, uncovered, until flesh just flakes with a fork, about 15 minutes. Serve garnished with basil leaves and lemon wedges.

Serves 2

{ Salmon in Bed with Fennel }

The sweet licorice flavor of the fennel and salmon are great bed-mates. Serve with pinot noir wine, roasted potatoes, and a green veg-etable or salad.

1 pound salmon fillet

1 small fennel bulb, trimmed and thinly sliced

2 tablespoons extra virgin olive oil

Salt and pepper to taste

Lemon wedges for garnish

1. Preheat oven to 500° F.

2. Pour 1 tablespoon of olive oil in a baking dish large enough to hold the salmon. Arrange fennel slices in bottom of pan.

3. Rub salmon with remaining tablespoon of olive oil and season with salt and pepper. Set salmon on top of fennel. Place fish in pre-heated oven. Lower temperature to 400° F and cook fish until opaque, about 20 minutes. Serve garnished with lemon wedges.

{ King Lapetamaka's Grilled shrimp }

Here's our version of this lusty dish. If you are short on time, substitute 1 cup of your favorite teriyaki sauce for our version. Serve with rice and sautéed or grilled vegetables.

1 (16 ounce) can pineapple chunks

1 cup teriyaki sauce (recipe follows)

1 pound extra large or jumbo shrimp, peeled and deveined

Bamboo skewers, soaked in water for 1 hour (the number of skewers needed will depend on the length of the skewers and size of the shrimp)

1. Drain pineapple, reserving the juice. In a medium-sized bowl, mix ½ cup of pineapple juice with teriyaki sauce. Place shrimp in a Ziploc bag or glass baking dish and combine with marinade. Refrigerate for at least 15 minutes and up to 1 hour.

2. Preheat grill on medium.

3. Thread 4 or 5 shrimp, alternating with pineapple chunks, onto two soaked bamboo skewers held slightly apart. (Using 2 skewers keeps the shrimp from rotating.)

4. Lightly oil the grill grate. Place shrimp/pineapple kebobs on grill and cover. Grill shrimp on one side just until they start to turn opaque around the edges, about 2 minutes. Turn shrimp and cook until shrimp are completely opaque and feel firm, about 2 additional minutes.

{ Teriyaki sauce }

½ cup soy sauce

¼ cup sherry

¼ cup dark sesame oil

1 tablespoon grated gingerroot

2 garlic cloves, minced

2 tablespoons honey

Combine all ingredients in a small bowl and refrigerate until ready to use.

{ The cooking couple's clambake }

This dish is adapted from a recipe created by *New York Times* columnist Mark Bittman, and is truly the easiest and best version of a clambake that we have ever made.

1 tablespoon fennel seeds (optional)

½ pound smoky slab bacon (optional)

12 hard-shell clams

2 pounds mussels, washed and debearded

1 pound new potatoes, cut into quarters

2 live lobsters (1¼ to 1½ pounds each)

2 ears corn, shucked

Melted butter (as much as you like)

1. In the bottom of a big, deep pot large enough to hold all of the ingredients (basically, the largest stock pot you own; nineteen-inch lobster pots are perfect for this), place the fennel seeds and bacon. Add the clams and mussels, followed by the potatoes. Place the lobsters and corn on top of the potatoes.
2. Add ½ a cup of water, cover the pot, and turn heat to high.
3. Let clambake cook, shaking pot occasionally, for 20 minutes. Remove lid, being careful not to burn yourself, and check a potato to see if it is tender. If potato is still hard, cook for an additional 5 to 10 minutes.
4. Remove all ingredients with tongs and set on a very large platter. Serve with melted butter for dipping.

Serves 2

{ Passionate Paella }

This is one of the first dishes Michael used to woo Ellen, and it's still one of our favorites. While it contains many ingredients, paella is easy to make and is great for leftovers.

¼ cup olive oil

2 pounds chicken pieces (legs, thighs, breasts, and/or wings)

1 medium onion, chopped

1 red bell pepper, diced

1 green bell pepper, diced

5 cups chicken stock or canned low-sodium chicken broth

4 garlic cloves, minced

3 cups short-grain rice

1 teaspoon salt

½ teaspoon black pepper

1 teaspoon paprika

6 strands saffron

4 tomatoes, diced

½ pound large shrimp, peeled and deveined

24 clams or mussels

1 cup peas

8 canned artichoke hearts

¼ cup fresh parsley, chopped

1. In large casserole or paella pan, heat oil over medium heat. Add chicken pieces and cook until brown on all sides. Remove chicken and set aside.

2. Add onion and peppers to the pan and sauté for 5 minutes.

3. In a separate pot, bring chicken stock or broth to a boil.

4. Add garlic and rice to onions and peppers, and sauté for another minute.

5. Reduce heat to low and add salt, pepper, paprika, saffron, tomatoes, boiled stock, and cooked chicken pieces to pan. Cover and cook for 25 minutes. Check casserole occasionally. If rice appears too dry add more stock or water at any point. (The rice should be moist, not soupy.)

6. Stir in shrimp, cover, and cook for 5 minutes.

7. Add clams or mussels, peas, and artichoke hearts and cook until the mollusks open, about 4 minutes. Sprinkle with parsley. Stir gently to combine ingredients, and serve.

Serves 4

{ Chef Joho's Famous Shrimp Bag }

This recipe comes from Brasserie Jo, our favorite French brasserie, located in Boston and Chicago. It's a bit challenging but worth the effort. Serve with diced tomatoes and scallions, and French bread.

6 tablespoons butter

1 leek, washed, trimmed, and sliced

1 cup sliced mushrooms

½ cup red and green bell peppers, chopped

8 ounces medium shrimp, peeled

Salt and pepper to taste

6 sheets phyllo dough

¼ cup bread crumbs

1. Preheat over to 350° F.
2. In a large sauté pan, melt 2 tablespoons butter over medium-low heat. Sauté mushrooms, leek, and peppers until soft, about 10 minutes.
3. Add shrimp and sauté until cooked through, about 5 additional minutes. Season with salt and pepper.
4. Melt remaining 4 tablespoons of butter. Spread the butter with a brush on 1 sheet of phyllo dough. Sprinkle with about 1 teaspoon of bread crumbs. Repeat 2 additional times stacking the phyllo on top of each other for a total of 3 layers of phyllo.
5. Using a sharp knife, cut stacked phyllo into 4 strips, place the 4 strips on a cutting board, and fan out into the shape of a star.
6. Place half the sautéed leek, mushroom, pepper, shrimp mixture in the center of the phyllo dough star. Bring the 8 ends of the star to the center to form a bag, and twist together. Repeat steps 3 through 5 using remaining phyllo and shrimp mixture.
7. Bake in preheated oven until crisp, about 25 minutes.

Aphrodite Aphro-snacks

{ ultimate vodka cocktail sauce }

Serve this sauce, which is chock-full of aphrodisiacs, with large cocktail shrimp placed in a martini glass, or with grilled scallops and/or shrimp.

¼ cup vodka

½ cup tomato sauce

2 teaspoons grated horseradish

Dash Tabasco or other hot sauce

1 garlic clove, minced

Salt and pepper to taste

Combine ingredients in a small bowl and chill until ready to serve.

{ caviar indulgence }

Enjoy this decadent spread with plenty of champagne or ice-cold vodka.

2 hard-boiled eggs, peeled and chilled

¼ cup chopped parsley

1 medium red onion, finely chopped

½ cup sour cream

Lemon wedges

4 ounces smoked salmon

Blinis (see recipe page 90)

½ cup sour cream

2 ounces (or more) caviar

1. Separate hard-boiled egg yolks from whites. Chop each separately.
2. Warm blinis and place sour cream in a bowl.
3. Place chopped yolks and whites, parsley, red onion, and smoked salmon around the rim of an elegant serving dish in small mounds. Place caviar in the center of the dish.
4. Top warm blinis with sour cream and caviar and any of the other ingredients on the serving dish that you would like.

{ Elegant Eggs }

Serve with champagne or mimosas and toasted white bread for a light and elegant brunch.

2 eggs

1 ounce caviar

1. Cook eggs (soft-boil) in boiling water for 4 minutes, no more! Place eggs in egg cups (if you do not have egg cups, shot glasses or sake cups work nicely), remove tops of eggs with a sharp knife, and sprinkle eggs with caviar.

Serves 2

4

chiLe Peppers:
The Aphrodisiac Dominatrix

Come on, baby, light my fire, come on, baby, light my fire
Try to set the night on fire. . . .

–Jim Morrison, The Doors

There's a fine Line between pleasure and pain, and chile peppers straddle the divide like a dominatrix dishing out both in equal measure. With a flick of her whip she'll bring you from the depths of hell to the heights of ecstasy and back again, laughing all the while, as she flogs your taste buds—and libido—into a fiery fury.

The heat in chile peppers ignites your senses, triggering a series of physical reactions that resemble sexual arousal. You sweat. Your lips tingle and burn. Your heartbeat and metabolism increase. Skin flushes. The burning sensation of biting into chile-laden cuisine creates a state of euphoria similar to the endorphin rush experienced after an orgasm. Love hurts, and chile peppers hurt sooooooo good!

A dose of heat in the form of fiery foods can catapult your palate and sex life out of the frying pan and into the fire. For The Cooking Couple, cuisine made with hot peppers begins a chain reaction that ends with combustible sex. Olé! Maybe that's one reason chile peppers turn up the heat for roughly a quarter of the planet's population—about 1.3 billion people. In countries where chiles play a major culinary role, a meal without fire is like sex without an orgasm.

HOW HOT IS HOT?

The heat of chile peppers is rated by an index called Scoville units, developed in 1912 by Detroit pharmacist Wilbur Scoville.

Initially, the system used human testers to measure the heat in peppers. Scoville mixed ground chile peppers with sugar water and had a group of tasters sip the mixture in increasingly diluted concentrations until they could no longer detect the capsaicin, a powerful, flavorless, odorless chemical that makes chile peppers hot. A number was assigned to each chile pepper based on how much it needed to be diluted so that tasters could no longer feel the burn.

While Scoville units are still used today, the heat is measured by a more sophisticated process called liquid chromatography, not the taste buds of mere mortals. Peppers range in Scovilles from 0 for an ordinary bell pepper to 350,000 to 577,000 for the red Savina habañero, the world's hottest pepper. Pure capsaicin measures 15 million to 16 million Scoville units.

The heat in chiles tends to be concentrated in the interior veins and the seeds. How hot a pepper gets depends on a number of factors. In general, the more mature the pepper, the more capsaicin it contains. Dry, hot, sunnier climates tend to produce the hottest peppers. Cooler, wetter, cloudier climates produce wimpier varieties even when using similar seeds. With the exception of the habañero—a relatively large pepper and one of the hottest—smaller peppers tend to be more fiery than their larger siblings.

No one is certain why physical pain arouses some people, but there are several theories. Pleasure centers in the body and receptors in the brain are closely linked to pain centers in the body and brain. In some people, nerves that transmit pain can become crosswired with nerves that convey pleasure. This may be one reason some people are sexually aroused (in some cases to the point of orgasm) by spanking. It is theorized that the nerves running from the genitals to the brain are closely coupled to the nerves in the buttocks, so stimulating the buttocks leads to sexual arousal and pleasure for some.

Pain also triggers the release of endorphins, natural pain-killers with a similar chemical structure to morphine that are connected to the brain's pleasure centers. (The word *endorphin* comes from "endogenous morphine.") Endorphins, discovered in the heat of the 1970s sexual revolution, are believed to influence appetite control and the pituitary gland's release of sex hormones. Enjoyable, sensory experiences (including making love and eating delicious foods) raise endorphin levels, resulting in a natural high that creates a craving for another endorphin rush that can be satisfied only by more pleasure. That's why you want another orgasm after great sex and another dish after the first bowl of ice cream. Endorphins are so powerful that drugs that block them can actually stop compulsive eaters from bingeing.

Endorphins are also responsible for another famous type of high, called "chile head." Capsaicin irritates trigeminal nerve cells, pain receptors lining the mouth, nose, and throat, which results in a burning sensation. Your body's nerves respond to the stimulation by sending pain messages to the brain. The brain receives the signals just as it would for a real burn and reacts by releasing endorphins, which in excess produce a feeling of euphoria similar to runners' high. Not only does eating chile peppers spark the release of endorphins, capsaicin also increases mouth sensitivity and makes food tastier and more flavorful.

Scientists are starting to prove what folk healers and ancient cultures have known all along: Chile peppers and their active chemical, capsaicin, are valuable additions to our modern medical arsenal.

Over 2,000 studies have been done on chile peppers, revealing that capsaicin can help numb pain, especially arthritis, and may decrease the risk of heart disease and stroke by reducing cholesterol and preventing blood clots.

Dr. David Ziment of the University of California in Los Angeles

sex, god's analgesic

Wondering why sex brings pleasure and relieves pain? Sex, particularly sensual touch, triggers the secretion of oxytocin, a hormone that induces pleasurable sensations, plays a role in sexual performance, and encourages us to bond with our lover. Oxytocin, which increases three- to fivefold during orgasm, causes the release of endorphins, which create the feeling of euphoria experienced during and after climax. The high levels of endorphins triggered by sexual pleasure act as an analgesic, temporarily relieving pain.

If she's complaining about cramps, give her nature's Midol—an orgasm. The next time your partner says, "Not tonight, dear, I have a headache," offer to give him or her an erotic massage that will send oxytocin into the bloodstream.

The key to erotic massage is to bring your partner to a high level of arousal and let him or her float there before orgasm. Follow these steps:

1. *Set the stage.* Turn up the heat so the room is warm and comfortable. Turn off the phone. Dim the lights, play sensual music, and perhaps heat some aromatherapy oil.

2. *Make your partner comfortable.* Have him or her lie down on a bed or the floor, cradled or supported by a few pillows. Have blankets available if it's cool.

3. *Lubrication:* To minimize friction between your hands and your partner's body, use a good lubricant to make the experience more pleasurable. (We know this is the chile chapter, but chile oil is *not* appropriate.) Water-, oil-, and silicone-based lubricants are fine for most body parts, but if you are massaging a woman's genitals, use water-based lubricants only. (Other lubricants can cause vaginal infections.) You can purchase massage oil or use a light vegetable oil such as canola, soybean, or safflower, perhaps scented with a few drops of essential oils or our favorite, vanilla.

4. *Communicate.* During all phases of the massage, encourage requests and feedback about what types of strokes feel best. Be sensitive and stay connected.

5. *Basic body strokes.* Take your time and keep your hands somewhere on your partner's body at all times. Start with longer gliding strokes and proceed to deeper ones. Explore his or her whole body—back, legs, feet, chest, arms, hands, and face.

6. *Genital exploration.* Once you've massaged your partner's body and he or she is relaxed, you can engage in genital massage. Start by slowly teasing the inner thighs, pubic region, and genitals. Stay tuned in to your partner's wants, desires, and moans. Let your partner know that massaging him or her is a powerful aphrodisiac for you as well.

has referred to hot peppers as "Nature's Robitussin" because chiles can relieve bronchitis and coughs, as well as a host of illnesses including asthma, headaches, and arthritis. Researchers at Yale University School of Medicine have invented a hot chile pepper candy that decreases mouth pain in cancer patients on chemotherapy.

Just as studying morphine led to the discovery of nerve pathways in the brain that suppress pain, according to David Julius and Michael Caterina of the University of California in San Francisco, discovering the target of capsaicin activity will help clarify how pain is produced.

All from a little pepper.

While chile peppers are not physically addictive in the way that some drugs and alcohol can be, the true chile head quickly becomes addicted to the next endorphin high. But in order to reach a state of euphoria, he must seek hotter and hotter horizons, because it takes spicier peppers in larger doses to reach the next pleasure plateau. That's one reason an entire industry has been born to provide these folks with their next fix.

substance P:
The Madame X of the Aphrodisiac world

A mysterious chemical called substance P desensitizes your reaction to hot peppers. This exotic beauty is a neurotransmitter found in nerve cells, as well as in the brain, spinal cord, and intestines. When you eat hot peppers, the capsaicin in the chiles causes the nerve cells in the spinal cord to release substance P, which signals the brain that you are in pain. But as you eat more peppers your nerve cells become more sensitive to substance P and less likely to transmit pain messages to the brain.

So, the more heat you eat, the more heat you need to reach satisfaction. P is for pleasure, P is for pain. Aphrodisiacs' femme fatale, don't forget her name.

Global warming

Chile peppers have been valued for centuries around the globe for their ability to arouse. Wondering why Szechuan- and Hunan-style Chinese dishes can be so hot and spicy? It's because in China, chile peppers are considered to be a potent sexual stimulant and are therefore used freely in the cuisine.

In Guadeloupe, chile peppers are known as "le derriere de Madame Jacques" (in English, "the rear of Madame Jacques"). We have no idea what the significance of this reference is other than Madame Jacques must have had a pretty nice butt. The natives make a potent aphrodisiac punch by combining chile peppers with crushed peanuts, cinnamon, nutmeg, brandied vanilla beans, and a locally produced liqueur, crème de banana. This odd-sounding concoction is actually surprisingly tasty. And it works!

{ Madame Jacques's Pepper Punch }

2 jalapeño, serrano, or habañero chile peppers, chopped
1 cup sugar
2 tablespoons crushed peanuts
¼ teaspoon cinnamon
Pinch of nutmeg
½ brandied vanilla bean (see recipe page 67)
4 ounces crème de banana

1. Mix peppers with sugar and 1 cup water.
2. In small saucepan bring pepper/sugar mixture to a boil, then lower heat and simmer until mixture is reduced to about ½ cup and resembles a thin syrup, about 30 minutes. Strain mixture through cheesecloth or strainer and let cool. (Try syrup on ice cream, or in mixed drinks such as mint julep as a substitute for regular "simple syrup." Store syrup in a covered jar in the refrigerator.)
3. In a blender blend 2 tablespoons pepper/sugar syrup, peanuts, cinnamon, nutmeg, vanilla bean, and crème de banana with 2 cups ice. Strain, and serve in a goblet while toasting Madame Jacques.

Serves 2

A Hot Time in the Old Town Tonight

Over the last ten years, the fiery foods industry has grown by nearly 50 percent and is estimated to be worth about $2.5 billion a year. Salsa outsells ketchup; southwestern food is popular from New Mexico to New England; and hot sauces with wild names like Nuclear Hell, After Death, Capital Punishment, Last Rites, and Endorphin Rush are sold everywhere. There are Web sites, cultlike groups, gatherings, magazines, and festivals devoted to chile peppers. It's a culinary global warming!

In some cultures chiles are believed to have magical powers. The Inca Indians of Panama tied a string of chiles together behind their boats to repel sharks and ward off other evils lurking in the water. The Colorado Indians of the Amazon burned chile peppers in an open fire and ate them to ward off *luban oko* (the red demon), who the natives believed drank its victims' blood. During warrior initiation rites, the Carib people of the Caribbean rubbed chile juice into the wounds of youths. What fun! Makes studying for your bar mitzvah or communion seem pretty wimpy by comparison.

Because of the passion that chiles inflame, they have been banned by everyone from the clergy to government and school administrators. In the 1970s the Peruvian government declared hot chile sauce an aphrodisiac and banned it from prison food, declaring it inappropriate "for men forced to live a limited lifestyle" because it could "arouse their sexual desire."

Observing how passionate the natives were about hot peppers, José de Acosta, a Jesuit priest and historian, expressed a concern in 1590 about chile peppers. He believed the peppers were an aphrodisiac and warned Spanish colonists in Mexico and Peru not to eat them. Of course this only made chiles more popular among the adventurous newcomers, many of whom had native servants or wives who introduced them to the power and pleasures of hot, spicy food.

Closer to home, chiles and other highly spiced foods were taboo on the menu in many convent schools because administrators felt hot foods led to loose behavior. Incidentally, hot dogs, an obvious phallic food, were often served cut up to keep the young ladies from having lewd thoughts. The nuns should have banned mustard, which has a long history as an aphrodisiac both topically and internally and is still believed by some to stimulate sexual activity by triggering the release of sex hormones. To boost his masculinity, Frederick the Great regularly drank a mixture of mustard, coffee, and champagne, and hot mustard baths were used to increase libido in women.

The Aphrodisiac condiment

Credit for popularizing hot cuisine goes partially to the McIlhenny family of Louisiana, who have tirelessly plugged their Tabasco Pepper Sauce since its invention in 1868. The concentrated sauce, which was meant to be sprinkled, not poured, was initially sold in discarded cologne bottles decorated with homemade labels. The sauce was patented in 1870 and quickly became popular throughout the United States and England. Along with the original patented Tabasco Pepper Sauce, there is now a Tabasco Green Pepper Sauce, a Garlic Pepper Sauce, and a Habañero Pepper Sauce.

They also sell a Bloody Mary mix. The original Bloody Mary was invented by American bartender Fernand Petiot at Harry's New York Bar in Paris during the 1920s. In 1934, Petiot started working at the King Cole Bar at the St. Regis in New York. He continued to mix his Bloody Marys, but he started to spike them with black pepper, cayenne pepper, Worcestershire sauce, lemon, and a generous splash of Tabasco for patrons who liked their drinks, and amour, on the hot side.

variety is the spice of life

It doesn't matter who you are, or what you've done, or think you can do. There's a confrontation with destiny awaiting you. Somewhere, there is a chile you cannot eat.

–Daniel Pinkwater, "A Hot Time in Nairobi"

There are hundreds of chile pepper varieties, ranging widely in size, shape, color, taste, and heat. Here are some of the most popular.

Anaheim: 1,000 scovilles

Virgins start here.

Also known as the New Mexico chile, this pepper is six to seven inches long. Don't let his size scare you. He's really very tender and sensitive, with a sweet flavor that works well in salsas and soups. Red when ripe, Anaheims are often dried and used for ornamental purposes.

Ancho: 1,000 scovilles

The chocolate lover's chile.

The ancho is three to six inches long and turns red to brown when mature. It has a sweet, raisin-like flavor perfect for sauces, stews, or purées. The ancho is often sold dried and used in traditional Mexican mole sauce, which is made with chocolate. An aphrodisiac double eagle!

cascabel: 3,000 scovilles

Mild yet wild.

This round, dark-reddish chile has a deep, rich, nutty flavor that is excellent in sauces, stews, soups, and salsas. Add a little cascabel pepper to ordinary tomato sauce to give it a kick.

jalapeño: 2,500 to 5,000 scovilles

Mercury rising.

Raise the heat and smoke these babies for a chipotle good time. Jalapeños are two inches long and half an inch wide, versatile, and hot. Use them in sauces, salsas, and bean dishes. The mature pepper is red or purplish black, and when smoked it is known as a chipotle. Remember, drying turns the heat up tenfold.

GuajiLLo: 5,000 scoviLLes

A divine gift from the chile gods.

One of the holy trinity of peppers used in moles, these babies are heaven-sent. The guajillo is a dried chile that measures four to six inches. A favorite in Mexican cooking, the ripened chile is brownish red in color and has a sweet berry flavor that is great in stews and sauces. Transform plain, boring pasta dishes into something extraordinary by adding sautéed guajillos to sauces. Also great in pesto.

serrano: 5,000 to 15,000 scoviLLes

Silken heat to a tango beat.

Earthy and sweet, serranos will serenade your lover's taste buds with a smooth yet intense warmth that tickles palate and passion equally. Also known as chile verde, this ½-inch-long, ½-inch-wide pepper is red when mature, dries very well, and is also delicious roasted. Great in sauces, salsas, soups, and stews.

Japone: 25,000 scoviLLes

Taste bud hari-kari.

Can you say "otsunaaji"? That's Japanese for "spicy." The japone has been heating up passion in the Orient for centuries. This red chile is two to three inches long and has a real kick that adds heat to whatever it touches. A staple in Asian dishes from stir-fries to peanut sauces.

penis pepper: 30,000 to 40,000 scoviLLes

Yes, that's what he looks like.

This very hot Latin lover likes to brag about his size and heat. (What man doesn't?) Measuring up to six inches long on a good day, he is yellow or red when ripe, has little flavor (but lots of heat), and is mainly dried and used for decoration.

Thai: 50,000 to 100,000 Scovilles

Thai yourself down.

This little beauty is going to blast you from home to Bangkok and back again. Also known as the red Amazon, this small pepper (it is one-half to one inch long) is red when mature and has a heat that sticks with you long after the meal. Frequently used in Asian cooking, it's great in stir-fries, soups, and stews.

Macho Green/Macho Red: 75,000 to 100,000 Scovilles

You're in the big leagues now, boys!

They might be called macho but the real question is, are you? This lilliputian pepper is one-quarter to half an inch long and has a bite like an angry Chihuahua. Add to salsas, soups, and stews. A little goes a long way.

Jamaican Hot: 50,000 to 100,000 Scovilles

"Jah, man, dees peppers be a' smokin'."

Roll one up and check out de buzz. "No women, no cry. I got my chile high." Jamaican hots are red and fat and measure about an inch in length. Try them in classic Caribbean dishes such as Jamaican jerk and keep a Red Stripe handy.

Habañero: 100,000 to 300,000 Scovilles

This ain't no party, this ain't no disco, this ain't no foolin' around.

Handle with extreme caution! These babies are hot!! Habañeros are a powerful, flavorful round chile with a slight citrus zing. They vary in color from green when unripened to red when fully developed. Habañeros are delicious eaten fresh in salsas spiked with a little lime. They pair beautifully with tropical and citrus fruits, so toss them into a fruit salsa or try our recipe for Hot Mango Ice Cream on page 139. C'mon, be brave. The heat of these chiles is intense, but it does dissipate rapidly.

savina Habañero: 350,000 to 570,000 scoviLLes

For thrill-seeking death freaks only!

The Heavyweight Chile Champion of the World. These peppers are enthroned in the *Guinness Book of World Records* as the world's hottest pepper. These bright red, round peppers are patented and grown in limited amounts by and under license

Nature's Fire Extinquisher

Many remedies, including water, milk, sugar, bread, beer, tomato juice, citrus fruit, and soda, have been proposed to cool chile's burn. The problem is that capsaicin binds with nerve receptors and is not easily dislodged. The antidotes are alcohol and fat, not water.

If you overdo the habañeros your best bet is to reach for regular full-fat dairy products, which contain casein, a protein that breaks capsaicin's hold on your mouth's pain receptors, and fat, which helps dissolve the capsaicin. Order a lassi (a popular Indian shake made from yogurt frequently flavored with herbs, spices, and fruit) or raita (a thick yogurt salad served as an accompaniment for hot Indian food) with that lamb vindaloo. Eat some sour cream or jack cheese with your fiery salsa, drink a glass of milk, or have a dish of good ol' ice cream.

A nice cold beer, which complements spicy food much better than milk, also does the trick because the alcohol in beer dissolves the capsaicin.

from GNS Spices. You must be a certified chile head (or just plain certifiable) to eat these. God be with you.

A Short, Hot History of Chile Peppers

Chile peppers, like chocolate, vanilla, avocados, and so many other aphrodisiacs, originated in the tropical regions of the New World. (Those Meso-Americans sure knew how to party.)

Excavations at Tehuacan (present-day southeastern Mexico) show that the native people living in the area started picking and eating chiles around 7000 B.C. and began cultivating them about 3,500 years later. After corn, chiles were probably the most important food to native cultures and responsible for much of the uniqueness of authentic Mexican cuisine.

Pre-Columbian civilizations showed their love and reverence for the plant by decorating everything from pottery to clothing with images of chile pods. Chile peppers were used to pay tribute to kings, and the Mayas, Incas, and Aztecs all offered chile peppers to their gods. The Aztecs were fond of the spicy erect fruit and added chile peppers to their chocolate, turning the drink into a doubly potent love food.

Columbus discovered chile peppers on his first voyage in 1492 on the island of Haiti, known at the time as Hispaniola. Thinking he was in India, Columbus called chiles "pimiento," the same name for the common spice black pepper, which was what Columbus was seeking. From the Americas, chile peppers quickly captured palates in Asia, India, Brazil, Africa, the Middle East, and Europe.

Today chiles still define Mexican and southwestern food to such an extent that the official state question of New Mexico, which produces more chile peppers than any other state, is "Red or green?" Chiles, that is. With chiles being such a powerful aphrodisiac, maybe the New Mexico state question should be "Your place or mine?" Now *that* would look cool on a license plate. Certainly better than "The Corn State" (Iowa).

some Don't Like it Hot

Mayan warriors blinded and stunned their enemies by hurling chile bombs at them. Today, capsaicin makes a great animal repellent and has been used to keep elephants, who have a keen sense of smell and dislike the fragrance of chile peppers, from wandering off wildlife reserves.

Chile pepper sprays are useful for keeping dogs, cats, and rodents out of garbage and for preventing squirrels from raiding the bird feeder. For you organic gardeners, try a chile pepper spray on your crops to keep deer, Peter Rabbit, and other pesky creatures from eating your summer bounty.

Americans have been slow in warming our palates and overcoming our bland, puritanical tongues. Chili powder, typically a blend of dried chiles, cumin, oregano, and sometimes black or red pepper and garlic powder, was invented in Texas over a hundred years ago but didn't become popular nationally until after World War II.

Fortunately, interest in and travel to places where chiles rule, an increase in immigration from Latin American and Asian countries, and the introduction of spicy foods in American restaurants have helped to put chiles on the culinary map.

The interest in healthy, low-fat food has also given chiles a boost. Folks are discovering that chiles add flavor to otherwise bland but healthy foods such as tofu, broccoli, and pasta, and they are satisfying, yet low in calories and fat and high in vitamins A and C. By weight, hot peppers contain over 350 percent more vitamin C than oranges.

Fire Kills

According to the journal *Toxicon,* if you weigh 140 pounds or less, drinking a quart and a half of Louisiana-style hot sauce will cause respiratory failure and kill you.

cooking with Fire

In many countries, chiles are eaten fresh and whole, diced and used as a garnish, or ground and added to cooked dishes. The best way to whip your chiles into shape and control the heat, flavor, and color that they add to dishes is to make them into purées (which will keep for a week in the refrigerator and up to six months in the freezer) and add them in small amounts to achieve the desired taste and heat.

To make a purée, wash several chiles and remove the stem and seeds. (Remember to use gloves when working with chiles.) Then purée in a blender or food processor. For a hotter condiment, purée some of the seeds with the flesh.

other uses for chiles

1. *Roasting:* Fresh chiles can be roasted until they blister over a gas flame or on an outdoor grill, which gives them a wonderful smoky flavor. After roasting, chiles should be cooled in a paper bag or wrapped loosely in foil to allow the skin to loosen and steam off. Roasted chiles can be stuffed, sliced into strips, or diced and frozen for future use.
2. *Sautéing:* Small, fresh chiles with tender skins can be diced, cut into pieces, or left whole and sautéed for five to ten min-

caution! HandLe with care
or don't HandLe at aLL!

Chile peppers are an aphrodisiac only when eaten. Capsaicin can cause painful burns, especially in sensitive areas like the eyes and genitals. There is actually a condition known as chile-willie ("willie" being the British term for "penis"), or hunan-hand in China, which occurs when a guy handles chiles and forgets to wash his hands thoroughly before relieving himself. (Yes, this is the one time it makes sense to wash your hands well *before* going to the bathroom.) The sensation that is so pleasurable in the mouth is very painful in the private parts. (It's also a very effective contraceptive, putting "willie" out of action for the rest of the evening.) Ditto when you touch your nose or eyes, which frequently occurs if you wear contact lenses. Practice safe chile handling. Wear rubber gloves or wash your hands thoroughly after working with them.

utes, or added directly to soups, stews, and sauces. Large chiles should be peeled before sautéing as the skin can be bitter and tough.

3. *Dried:* Dried chiles are a welcome addition to any passion pantry and tend to have a deeper, earthier flavor than fresh chiles, often with notes of smoke or fruit. You can buy dried chiles in most supermarkets. They should be soaked for at least twenty minutes before using to optimize flavor and texture. Remember, once they are soaked they should be handled carefully, just like fresh chiles. They can then be made into a purée or used directly in dishes. In general fresh chiles get milder when cooked, while dried chiles get hotter. The best rule of thumb is to add a little heat at a time until you reach the desired intensity.

Looking for Love in ALL the Hot Places

Don't have a red-hot lover? Try looking for lust wherever hot sauce is sold. Ladies, if you want to marry a millionaire (or at least a guy with a good income), your best bet for finding Mr. Right might just be looking for a guy who loves fiery food. According to fiery-foods.com, the average fiery foods consumer is male, between thirty-five and fifty-five, generally has a high-energy, risk-taking personality, and tends to earn at least $60,000 per year.

You can find Mr. Hot Times by attending one of the numerous chile festivals that take place across the country, such as the National Fiery Foods & Barbecue Show in Albuquerque, New Mexico; the Oxnard Salsa Festival in Oxnard, California; or the Florida Fiery Foods & Barbecue Show in St. Petersburg, Florida. Not only will you find an astonishing variety of hot and spicy foods to sample, from salsas and barbecue sauces to nuts, jams, candies, and chips; you'll also find a very favorable ratio of hot, hunky guys to gals.

Can't make it to a fiery food show? How about joining the Transcendental Capsaicinophilic Society, a new cult devoted to "the worship of all chiles; lifelong dedication to chile consumption, and making fun of people who just can't take that spicy food." Yes, they refer to themselves as a cult, but don't worry, they only wear saffron robes for special holidays like National Chile Month.

In her quest to find a "hot guy," a good friend of ours ran the following personal ad:

Come on, baby, light my fire!

Single, fiery female with hankering for habañeros seeks chile head with a well-hung jalapeño for hot, tasty times.

The response was overwhelming. She's now happily married to a skydiving, chile head lawyer with a good income and a generous jalapeño.

Need to add a little adventure to your mundane existence? Don't wait for lightning to strike. Grab a bunch of habañeros, jalapeños, or serranos tonight. Then show your lust object how to turn up the heat a few Scoville units and bow to the aphrodisiac dominatrix of pleasure and pain.

Lick the whip and let chiles free your libido and ignite your heart.

The cooking couple's chile pepper menu for amour

{ jalapeño vodka }

This drink is great with another of our favorite aphrodisiacs, oysters. The vodka-pickled jalapeños also make a great garnish for oyster shooters.

2 cups plain vodka

1 ounce dry white vermouth

1 fresh jalapeño pepper, seeded and quartered

Place all ingredients in a glass jar. Shake well and let sit in the refrigerator for 2 days. Remove pepper and enjoy. *Nostrovia!*

{ chile oil }

One of our favorite ways to add fire to any recipe is to zap the finished dish with a drop of chile oil. Making your own chile oil is quick and easy. Best of all, you get to call the shots both in terms of the types of peppers you use and the level of heat you want. Chile oil gets hotter as it ages, will keep for about six months, and makes a great gift for a hot head.

⅓ cup dried hot chile peppers such as Anaheim, jalapeño, or Thai

1 cup vegetable oil (we like to use peanut or olive)

1. In a small saucepan, heat chile peppers and oil over low heat for about 10 minutes. Make sure oil does not smoke or bubble. Let cool.
2. Place mixture in a glass jar or cruet and store in a cool, dark place.

Makes 1 cup

{ caribbean crostini }

1 tablespoon olive oil

2 garlic cloves, minced

2 teaspoons Caribbean hot sauce

½ loaf French bread

2 tomatoes, sliced

1. Preheat toaster oven to 350° F.
2. Combine olive oil, garlic, and hot sauce.
3. Cut bread in half lengthwise and again cut in half in the middle of the loaf to make a total of 4 pieces. Spread the inside of each piece with the olive oil mixture and top with tomatoes. Bake until golden brown, about 5 minutes.

{ pad thai }

This dish works well as an appetizer or main course. Vary the hot sauce and roasted chiles to suit your taste. Look for fish sauce, rice noodles, and dried Thai chile peppers in Asian markets or the Asian section of your supermarket.

⅓ cup rice or white wine vinegar

3 tablespoons sugar

2 tablespoons hot sauce or to taste

2 tablespoons fish sauce (optional)

½ pound tofu, cut into cubes

2 tablespoons soy sauce

8 ounces rice noodles

2 tablespoons peanut or canola oil

2 eggs, beaten

4 scallions, cut into 1-inch lengths

½ pound medium cooked shrimp

3 cups bean sprouts

⅓ cup peanuts, chopped

Lime wedges for garnish

Dried, ground Thai chile peppers to taste, or your favorite Asian-style chile sauce

1. To make sauce, in a small bowl combine vinegar, sugar, hot sauce, and fish sauce. Set aside.

2. Mix tofu and soy sauce.

3. In a large saucepan, bring 3 quarts of water to a boil. Add rice noodles and cook until opaque, 5 to 6 minutes. Drain and rinse with cold water.

4. Heat a large skillet over medium heat. Add oil. When oil is hot, add eggs and stir continuously until firm. Add tofu and scallions and cook, stirring frequently, for another 3 to 4 minutes.

5. Rinse noodles again with cold water to separate. Drain well. Add noodles along with prepared sauce to skillet. Cook mixture, stirring often, until sauce is absorbed and noodles are heated through, 3 to 4 minutes. Stir in shrimp and cook for another minute. Stir in bean sprouts.

6. To serve, place individual portions of noodle mixture on plates. Sprinkle with chopped peanuts and chopped cilantro and garnish with lime wedges. Add ground Thai chile peppers or Asian chile sauce to bring dish to your personal heat preference.

Serves 4 as an appetizer, 2 as a main course

{ Chile Relleno Casserole }

A fun variation on chiles rellenos that avoids the hassle and calories of deep-frying. Cut the recipe in half and freeze one portion for a quick, romantic meal.

8 roasted Anaheim or New Mexico chiles, peeled and seeded

8 corn tortillas

1 cup cheddar or Monterey Jack cheese, grated

1 cup prepared salsa

1 cup sour cream or yogurt

1. Preheat oven to 350° F. Grease a 9x13-inch baking dish.
2. Cut open one roasted chile and place on top of one corn tortilla. Fill chile with 2 tablespoons cheese. Roll up tortilla and place in baking dish. Repeat for remaining tortillas.
3. Mix salsa and sour cream (or yogurt) and spoon mixture over tortillas.
4. Bake in preheated oven until sauce is bubbling and tortillas are just starting to brown, about 20 minutes.

Serves 8 as an appetizer, 4 as a main course

{ Fiery Steak Fajitas }

According to legend, cowboys devised this recipe as a way to make the skirt steak (which is a very tough cut of beef taken from the midsection, or "cummerbund," of the cow, called a *fajita* in Spanish) given to them on the trail tender and flavorful. This is great, sexy finger food for cowboys and cowgirls alike.

1 pound skirt or round steak, trimmed of fat and membrane

4 garlic cloves, peeled and minced

1½ teaspoons ground cumin

1 teaspoon dried oregano

1 fresh jalapeño pepper, diced

1 lime

Salt and freshly ground black pepper to taste

8 corn tortillas

Salsa and guacamole

1. Score the meat on both sides by making $\frac{1}{8}$-inch-deep slashes in the steak approximately an inch apart.
2. Combine garlic, cumin, oregano, and jalapeño pepper.
3. Rub the mixture all over the meat. (Don't forget the rubber gloves!) Place meat in a Ziploc bag and let marinate in the refrigerator, turning occasionally, for up to 24 hours.
4. Preheat grill to medium high. Squeeze the juice of the lime on both sides of the steak and sprinkle with salt and pepper.
5. Wrap tortillas in aluminum foil and place on a warm spot on the grill or in a toaster oven set at 250° F.
6. Grill the meat to suit your preference. (Personally, we recommend 3 to 4 minutes per side, per inch for a medium rare steak.) Place meat on a platter. Cover loosely with foil and let rest for 5 minutes.
7. Cut meat across the grain into diagonal strips. To serve, place several strips on the center of a corn tortilla along with salsa and guacamole. Roll up tortilla and enjoy.

Serves 4

Aphro-snacks

Once you become bit by the chile bug, there is no limit to the number of recipes you can zap with heat. Here are a couple of our favorite chile aphro-snacks.

{ HOT NUTS }

1 pound shelled nuts (You can use peanuts, mixed nuts, or a combination of both.)

2 tablespoons butter

1 teaspoon ground cumin

1 teaspoon garlic powder

1 teaspoon freshly ground black pepper

Ground dried chiles or cayenne pepper to taste (We recommend
    starting with 1 teaspoon.)

Salt to taste

1. Preheat oven to 250° F.
2. Melt butter in a large roasting or jelly roll pan in the oven. Add nuts,
   cumin, garlic powder, black pepper, chiles or cayenne pepper, and
   salt and stir well to coat nuts with spices. Cook, stirring every 10 to
   15 minutes, until nuts are golden brown, about 45 minutes.
3. Spread nuts on absorbent paper towels and let cool. Store in air-
   tight container.

{ Lite Chile Mix }

Feel free to vary the ingredients in the nut recipe in terms of both the
spices and the nuts. For example, for a lite, spicy mix, coat 3 cups air-
popped popcorn, 2 cups corn or rice Chex cereal, 2 cups pretzels, and
1 cup soy nuts with cooking spray, toss with spices, and bake in jelly
roll pan or baking dish at 250° F for 15 to 20 minutes.

{ Chile Chocolate Syrup }

For a simple, yet sensational dessert sauce with an aphrodisiacal
double edge, spike chocolate sauce (Good old Hershey's syrup will
do.) with ancho chile powder to taste. Pour over ice cream or use for
dipping strawberries and other fruits. (For an easy recipe for chocolate sauce, see page 73.)

{ Chocolate Chile Fondue }

For a richer chocolate fix, cover 2 dried habañero chiles with boiling
water and let sit for 20 minutes. Purée chiles in a blender or food
processor. Melt 2 ounces of dark chocolate in the microwave or in a
double boiler. Mix with chiles and use for dipping strawberries or other
fruits, nuts, and cookies.

{ HOT Mango Ice cream }

Habañero chile peppers have a citrus flavor that pairs beautifully with fruit. Here's a quick, easy, unusual dessert that will heat you up as it cools you down.

Cover 2 dried habañero chiles with boiling water and let sit for 20 minutes. In a blender or food processor purée chiles with one ripe mango. Fold into a pint of softened vanilla ice cream. Refreeze and enjoy.

5

Licorice and Its Kissing cousins (Inbreeding Allowed)

Our audience is like people who like licorice. Not everyone likes licorice, but the people who like licorice really *like licorice.*

—Jerry Garcia, The Grateful Dead

Chocolate is the silk of the candy world; black licorice is the leather. Dark, earthy, sexy, and mysterious, licorice is more than a little like the actor Samuel L. Jackson.

Prized for its sweetness and aphrodisiacal power, licorice traverses the divide between food, flavor, fragrance, and medicine. An aphrodisiacal rebel, licorice is untraditional and daring, but always fashionable. Black never goes out of style.

Licorice has even given chocolate a run for its money on the aphrodisiacal hit parade. The sweet, erotic root (which is generally crushed into a pulp and boiled with water to make a liquid or solid extract before being used as a flavoring or medicine) can boost sexual desire because it contains small amounts of phytoestrogens, plant chemicals that are similar to the female sex hormone estrogen. In addition, glycyrrhizin, the plant chemical found in licorice that makes it sweet, stimulates the production of hormones such as cortisone and aldosterone, and may one day be used to enhance the function of hormonal drugs.

The ancient Chinese, Egyptians, and Brahmans of India all used licorice to increase sexual arousal and stamina. More recently, sales of licorice skyrocketed in Germany, surpassing chocolate as a gift for lovers, as men discovered that Deutschland dames found licorice sexually arousing.

The Chinese still chew licorice root for sexual endurance, and the Hindus make a licorice tea with milk, honey, fennel juice, ghee (clarified butter), and sugar to boost sexual prowess. Herbalists often combine licorice root with other herbs, such as ginseng and saw palmetto, to protect the prostate gland and enhance erections for men, and balance hormones and reduce PMS in women.

You don't have to eat licorice to increase sexual desire. A whiff will do. Dabbing a little pastis, a licorice-flavored French cordial, or the licorice-flavored liqueur Pernod behind your ears can help fire up romance. According to Dr. Alan Hirsch, Director of the Smell and Taste Treatment and Research Foundation in Chicago, the smell of doughnuts paired with that of black licorice increased penile blood flow (a way to measure sexual arousal that involves placing a small blood pressure cuff around the penis) by over 30 percent. For women, the scents of Good & Plenty candy and cucumber increased vaginal blood flow by 13 percent. Among women who liked to masturbate, the combination of licorice candy scent and banana nut bread scent increased vaginal blood flow by a whopping 28 percent. How does a cucumber, Good & Plenty, banana nut bread sandwich sound?

Known as the "elixir of life," licorice and licorice candy have long been linked with lust. Early earth-based, mystical religions known as the Old Religion, Paganism, Wicca, or the Craft (which predate *Buffy the Vampire Slayer* by several thousand years), believed that Venus (the planet of love) and water (the element of emotions) ruled licorice. During the Middle Ages, witches were frequently consulted by lovelorn maidens and brokenhearted blokes in search of amorous lotions and elixirs. According to these pagan religions, licorice's dominant energy and magical uses were for love, sex, and fidelity, and licorice was therefore a common ingredient in passion potions and love brews.

Black licorice made from true licorice extract (look for it in health food stores) is a strong sexual stimulant when chewed. Try

Licorice Love Potion

To win the one you love or lust after, try the following magic potion:

By the light of a full moon on a night ruled by Venus, mix together one teaspoon licorice extract, 1/4 teaspoon dove's blood, three drops honey, and 7 rose petals. Stir with a green feather, and place seven drops in your love's grog. (This will be a bigger hit with your intended than Love Potion Number 9.)

To enhance the strength of your potion, light a red candle and repeat the following:

"For you I yearn.

For me you burn."

Visualize a night of romance with your love object while you conjure. (This shouldn't be too hard, since you can't stop thinking about him or her.)

Really dedicated to catching the one you love? Steal a lock of his or her hair. On the night of a new moon, braid it together with a lock of your own hair and a red ribbon. Tie the ends together to form a ring. Prick your finger, spill a drop of blood on the ring, and wear it until you've won him or her over.

When he or she comes to your house, put out a bowl of licorice candy and pop one into his or her mouth whenever you get a chance. If your plan works and you find yourself beside your beloved in the morning, serve our recipe for Arabic Egg Mash accompanied by champagne and Chocolate Fruit Salad.

munching a piece of licorice root while making your way to a sexy liaison with the one you love or lust after, and see what materializes. Better yet, share a few pieces with your lust object on a walk and see how long it takes to circle back to someone's abode for a little walk on the wild side!

Not a licorice lover yet? You may change your mind after you discover its ability to rev up romance. If you don't like one variety, try another! There's Italian, Kosher, sugar free, salted, grape, green apple, and mint; licorice babies, boats, cats, coins, jaw breakers, diamonds, white licorice popsicles, and our favorite, the licorice whip.

A Lick of Licorice

I bet you have on a thong made of licorice, don't you?

—Eddie Murphy as Buddy Love in
The Nutty Professor

The word *licorice* refers to both licorice candy and the licorice plant itself, a feathery-leaved, perennial herb native to the Mediterranean, central and southern Russia, and the area stretching from Asia Minor to Iran. Licorice still grows wild throughout parts of southern and central Europe, and is now widely cultivated throughout Europe, the Middle East, and Asia.

Licorice root is highly sought after for its sweetness, which is

Drink Like an Egyptian

The Coca-Cola of King Tut's day was a stimulating licorice beverage called *mai sus*. Here's our version of the ancient drink, which also contains anise seeds and honey, two other aphrodisiacs.

1 tablespoon sesame seeds
1 tablespoon anise seeds
2 licorice tea bags (Stash makes a very nice licorice tea.)
Honey to taste
Using a mortar and pestle or clean coffee grinder, grind the sesame and fennel seeds. Pour 2 cups of boiling water over tea bags and seeds and let steep for 5 minutes. Strain, and sweeten with honey to taste.

up to fifty times sweeter than sugar. Licorice's botanical name, *Glycyrrhiza,* given by the first-century Greek physician Diso-carides, comes from the Greek words *glukos* ("sweet") and *rizo* ("root").

Abundant, still-potent supplies of licorice were discovered in King Tut's tomb, and its first recorded use was written on Assyrian clay tablets dating back to 2500 B.C. Warriors chewed it to quench their thirst while on the march. Chinese Buddhist sages lauded licorice's valuable healing properties. The Roman scholar Pliny wrote that keeping a piece of licorice root in the mouth prevented hunger and thirst. Napoléon ate so much licorice during battle that his teeth turned black. (Ever see a picture of Napoléon smiling? Now you know why.) And Alexander the Great, the Scythian armies, and Caesar all gave licorice a hearty endorsement. Licorice was so popular in Europe that in 1305, Edward I of England taxed licorice imports to finance the repair of London Bridge. Which at the time was falling down. . . .

Millions of pounds of licorice root, mostly from the Mediterranean, are imported to the United States each year. (One licorice species is native to North America, but it isn't widely cultivated.)

Dem Bones

In the nineteenth century mummies were so common in Egypt that European travelers used them for fuel. But more discerning Egyptians ground them up and sold them as aphrodisiacs.

Perhaps mummy bones were considered to be an aphrodisiac because the ancient Egyptians were very open sexually. Much ancient Egyptian artwork depicts people engaged in sex. Single people, married couples, and even the gods had fun in bed. So much fun, in fact, that sex was also a key part of the afterlife. Male mummies had attached penises, female mummies had nipples, and many graves contained fertility dolls.

About 90 percent is used to flavor tobacco products (is this why Bogart and Bacall look so sexy smoking cigarettes and gazing into each other's eyes?), imbuing cigarettes, cigars, and pipe tobacco with a sweet, pleasant flavor. The extract taken from licorice root and the dried licorice root itself (both of which are very strong and can mask bad flavors) are also used to flavor food, candy, alcohol, cosmetics, and medicine. In Britain, licorice is used as an emulsifier to create foam in drinks, including alcoholic beverages. Anyone for a pint of licorice stout, mate?

Loving licorice is like learning to love fine, single-malt scotch. As your palate becomes more educated, you reach out for bolder and more unusual varieties, then suddenly you're hooked, searching gourmet food stores and the Internet for that perfect licorice buzz. True licorice is more intense and not as sweet as typical American licorice-type candy, which is usually flavored with antethole, a derivative of the anise plant (another aphrodisiac), and contains little or no real licorice. Real licorice has a rich, earthy, intense, smoky flavor that makes your taste buds stand up and salute.

Authentic licorice candy (made from water extracts of licorice root mixed with sugar, corn syrup, and flour) is far more popular in Europe, especially England, than in the States. Licorice got its start as a major player in the confectionery world in the early sixteenth century, when a group of monks in Pontefract, England (which today remains the center of the licorice confectionery industry and is still renowned for its licorice candy), started growing licorice root in their garden. Today licorice candy comes in over a dozen varieties, the roots varying in degrees of sweetness from mild to an almost sharp, peppery flavor, and in even more shapes and forms from ropes and laces to cream-filled sticks.

sexy ... and Dangerous

Like a raven-haired beauty in a dark café at midnight, licorice is sweet, sexy, seductive, and mysterious. But if you don't treat this lady right, she can be one dangerous dame. Just like a blonde in a Bond movie, licorice (yes, even the candy) can be toxic in large doses. (Remember Pussy Galore in *Goldfinger*?)

In the fifties, about a quarter of patients treated with licorice suffered side effects including water retention, headaches, abdominal pain, and shortness of breath. Initially, scientists thought the patients were allergic to licorice, but antihistamines (a medication used to treat allergic reactions) didn't help. Similar effects have also been reported by people who eat large quantities of licorice or use licorice-flavored tobacco products. The symptoms, which are caused by an excessive secretion of the hormone aldosterone, usually disappear when the licorice dosing is reduced or stopped.

Pregnant women, diabetics, and people with heart disease, high blood pressure, or severe menstrual disorders should all steer clear of large doses of licorice. If you fall into this category and are craving licorice, stick to sweets flavored with anise seed oil or just enjoy licorice's arousing aroma.

Just a spoonful of Licorice Helps the medicine go down

Licorice root has been prized for its medicinal properties for 5,000 years. It has been used therapeutically in both Western and Eastern medical systems and is one of the most extensively researched medicinal plants.

•In traditional Chinese medicine, licorice (called *gan cao*) is widely combined with other herbs to enhance their activity, reduce toxicity, and improve flavor. Its therapeutic uses include rejuvenating the heart and spleen, enhancing digestion (it's the

Asian version of Tums), and treating ulcers, colds, coughs, hepatitis, and skin disorders.

•In Europe, licorice has been used as a folk remedy for ulcers, and a drug made from licorice extract is now part of the standard treatment for gastric ulcers. The Europeans also add licorice to herbal formulas to prolong therapeutic effects and improve taste. The herb is also used to boost energy and the immune system and to treat arthritis and high cholesterol.

•Glycyrrhizin, the plant chemical that makes licorice sweet, is believed to increase hormone levels and prevent cancerous tumors, particularly of the colon and breast.

•The Teton Dakota Indians applied chewed licorice leaves to the backs of their horses to heal their sores. The root was also used in American folk medicine to treat toothaches, reduce fever, and help expel the placenta after childbirth.

Licorice's Kissing Cousins

An easy, tasty way to scent your life with licorice is to incorporate licorice's culinary cousins—fennel, anise, and star anise—into your diet. They all resemble licorice in flavor.

Anise (cultivated primarily for its seeds, which, along with its leaves, have a sweet, licorice flavor) and fennel belong to the same herb family as parsley, dill, cumin, carrot, and caraway, but not licorice. Star anise is the fruit of a small evergreen tree common to China and Japan called *Illicium verum.*

Fennel: The Orgy Seed

During Greek celebrations honoring Dionysus, the god of wine and fertility, people adorned themselves with crowns of fennel leaves and ate fennel seeds. These weren't just little parties where people sipped bad white wine and ate greasy hors d'oeuvres. We're talking bacchanalian orgies of lust where the hors d'oeuvres passed around were beautiful young maidens who represented the goddess of love and beauty, Aphrodite. Sexual intercourse was considered a form of worship. (Speak to your local priest, rabbi, minister, monk, imam, or ayatollah to get your conversion application.) This was stuff that even Mick Jagger could only dream about. Today, fennel still has a reputation as an aphrodisiac in many Mediterranean countries, particularly when used in fennel soup.

During the Middle Ages in Denmark, fennel was recommended to rejuvenate older men. (Could this be Mick's secret?) Fennel (*Foeniculum vaulgare,* known as finocchio, Florence fennel, common, and sweet fennel) refers to different parts of two similar plants, one used primarily as a vegetable, the other used for its seeds. The vegetable resembles celery on steroids and is grown mostly for its greenish-white, flattened bulb. The seeds of the other variety, common fennel, are used in Indian and Chinese spice mixtures and to flavor both savory and sweet dishes.

Like licorice, fennel is high in natural estrogen-like plant chemicals called phytoestrogens. These chemicals can help regulate hormone levels in women and may help stimulate menstruation and ease menopausal symptoms. In the 1930s, fennel was even investigated as a potential source of synthetic estrogen.

The vegetable fennel is rich in potassium (a mineral that has been found to help lower blood pressure), low in calories, and fat free, and has been used throughout history to alleviate hunger. Fennel is still regarded as an effective herb for weight loss because of its reputation as an appetite suppressant and an aid in the digestion of fat.

To keep their stomachs from grumbling, the Puritans munched on fennel seeds (nicknamed "meetin' seeds") during all-day church services. Apparently, no one told them that fennel was a potent aphrodisiac. Then again, who would? In those days, if you looked cross-eyed at a Puritan, they'd call you a witch, burn you at the stake, and then go back to torturing Indians in the name of God.

The ancient Greeks named fennel "marathon," from the word

Fennel seeds to the Rescue

Fennel seeds have been used to cure everything from snake and scorpion bites to hiccups, coughs, earaches, and toothaches. Here are some common fennel folk remedies.

- You've got a date, and bad breath. Chewing on a spoonful of fennel (or anise) seeds will freshen your mouth.
- Too much chow mein? Eat fennel or anise seeds to ease your tummy. The seeds aid digestion, which is why they are commonly served after Indian meals.
- The milk woman is late. Eating fennel seeds or drinking fennel tea seems to increase milk production in breast-feeding women. Anise seeds work in the same way.
- Can't sleep, don't count sheep. Instead, drink a cup of fennel or anise tea, which contain natural substances that help you sleep. According to folklore, sleeping on an anise-scented pillow will also prevent bad dreams.
- Time to warm your lover's body. Make a batch of Lover's Brew

{ Lover's Brew }

2 tablespoons fennel seeds

1 cup milk

1 tablespoon butter

2 tablespoons honey

2 tears (to induce crying without wreaking emotional havoc, we recommend slicing an onion)

2 cinnamon sticks

Boil the fennel seeds in ½ cup water. Strain and mix liquid with milk, butter, and honey. Cry on command and add tears to mixture. Heat until butter melts and serve in scarlet mugs garnished with cinnamon sticks.

maraino, which meant "to grow thin." The famous Battle of Marathon in 490 B.C. when the Persians invaded Greece was named Marathon because it was fought on a fennel field.

Fennel Fundamentals

When shopping for fennel look for compact, firm, blemish-free bulbs that are smooth and whitish-green, with the perky green stalks and leaves attached. (The leaves tend to wilt first. So healthy-looking greens mean the bulb is fresh as well.) To keep fennel fresh, cut the greens from the bulb, store them in separate plastic bags in the crisper drawer of the refrigerator, and use within three to four days.

In the raw, fennel is a refreshing palate cleanser that wakes up salads and the senses with its crunch and licorice-like flavor. The bulb flatters many other vegetables, pairs well with citrus fruits, and is a nice addition to an antipasto platter. (Simply slice fennel and serve with other raw vegetables, a little coarse salt for sprinkling, and a bowl of good-quality olive oil for dipping.)

Cooking tends to mellow fennel, softening its texture, sweetening its flavor, and taking away some of the licorice bite. Fennel bulbs are easy to prepare. Simply trim off the root end of the bulb, making sure not to cut all the way through the layers of the bulb so it stays together when sliced. Cut off the feathery stalk (save it for soups and stocks), and remove the thick, stringy, tough outer ribs. Cut the bulb in half, wash in cold water, and slice either horizontally or vertically as desired. It can be braised, caramelized, boiled, steamed, sautéed, grilled, and even fried.

The feathery foliage of both varieties looks like dill and is used as an herb to enhance soups, stocks, stews, and salads, and meat, fish, and pasta dishes. The French commonly add dried fennel branches to the fire when grilling fish while Italians braise or caramelize the fennel bulb, or serve it raw with a little lemon juice and olive oil. All the parts of both plants have varying degrees of fennel's characteristic gentle, sweet, warm licorice flavor.

Anise Essentials

Anise is a valuable tool for weaving culinary magic. Ruled by the planet Jupiter, the element air, and the energies of love, anise is still used magically as protection against evil and to flavor wedding cakes and ensure that the newly married couple's love will flourish. To promote love and help establish your relationship, try baking and eating some anise-flavored cookies.

Anise (*Pimpinella anisum umbelliferae*) was first used in ancient Egypt and is a bit stronger and sweeter than fennel. Anise, like fennel and licorice, has been used by humans in a wide variety of roles including as an aphrodisiac, and is still used as a powerful sexual stimulant in folk medicine.

The ancient Romans widely cultivated anise for its fragrance, flavor, and medicinal uses and baked special anise-flavored digestive cakes called *mustace.* It was considered so valuable that

{ Tipsy Gypsy }

Gypsies know a thing or two about love potions. Here's an old gypsy recipe using anise.

1 teaspoon anise extract

2 teaspoons wild oats*

1 cup Indian pennywort (also known as Gotu kola or Brahmi)

2½ cups vodka

6 dried apricots

Combine all ingredients. Place in a cool, dark place for 1 month. Strain. Store in the freezer and serve.

*There is something to the saying "sowing your wild oats." Wild oats are believed to be a sexual stimulant for both humans and animals. Oats are rich in many nutrients needed for sexual health, and some researchers believe oats balance hormone levels and make more testosterone available to the body, thus increasing libido. Hi ho Silver . . . away!

the citizens of Rome could pay their taxes in anise instead of cash. (Do not try this with the IRS. We did, we lost.)

Pythagoras, the sixth-century B.C. mathematician and philosopher, thought that holding anise could prevent epileptic seizures. (While it's easy to prove Pythagoras's theories on triangles, this one is a little harder to confirm.)

Hippocrates discovered a more plausible use for anise, to treat coughs. Anise was one of Emperor Charlemagne's favorite flavorings, a taste that he shared with mice, which during the sixteenth century were commonly baited with the licorice-scented plant.

Today, anise seeds are often added to rye bread and sweet baked goods and served, like fennel seeds, as an after-dinner nibble to aid digestion and combat bad breath. The oil of the anise seed is also used for cough remedies and to flavor licorice-like candies and liqueurs, including Greek ouzo, the French spirits pastis, Pernod, and anisette, as well as Benedictine and Boonekamp.

star anise

Like common anise, star anise tastes like licorice, is also used to flavor candy and food, and can be brewed into a fragrant tea. Medicinally, star anise has been used both as an aphrodisiac and as a stimulant, to improve alertness. It is known to decrease stress and enhance relaxation, sleep, emotional balance, and even your sense of humor. In the Amazon, star anise is thought to prevent fainting, and it is used to eliminate sad thoughts in menstruating women.

Also known as whole or Chinese anise, star anise is the hard, brown, star-shaped seed pod of a small evergreen tree that grows in southwestern China. Popular in Europe since the early 1600s, its flavor and fragrance resemble common anise seed, but star anise is more intense, robust, and licorice-like. It is an essential ingredient in Chinese five-spice powder (along with fennel seeds, Szechuan peppercorn, cinnamon, and cloves) and, like cinnamon bark, is widely used in braised dishes to give them a rich taste and fragrance. The star-shaped, warm spice has eight segments, each of which contain a seed, and is used to flavor teas, liqueurs, and stews as well as for tea-smoking (we know what you're thinking, and the answer is *no,* you don't roll it), a process that probably originated as a way to preserve food, but is now used to flavor dishes such as tea-smoked chicken.

Inbreeding Encouraged

When it comes to licorice recipes, inbreeding is encouraged. Try substituting the ground spices anise, fennel, and star anise for each other, or if you're really bold, try using Chinese five-spice powder instead of cinnamon, ginger, or nutmeg in baked fruit nut breads or spice cookies. (Bake a batch of five-spice powder cookies next Christmas and leave them for Saint Nick. We have it on good authority that Santa and Mrs. Claus really appreciate these aphrodisiac-laden treats.) You can find premixed Chinese five-spice powder in Asian supermarkets and natural foods stores, or you can make your own by mixing equal parts fennel seed, anise seed, Szechuan peppercorn, cinnamon, and cloves and grinding them in a clean blender or coffee bean grinder.

With so many ways to enjoy licorice-flavored foods, there's no excuse not to start incorporating licorice into your love life. You can start by sweetening each other's breath by nibbling a few fennel, anise, or star anise seeds. Toast your love with a French-inspired aperitif of Pernod or Anisette. Or simply cut up a fennel bulb and add it to your next vegetable platter. When you're ready to make licorice-flavored Cupid cuisine, you can move on to a fragrant bowl of fennel soup or a hearty, aphrodisiac-spiked bouillabaisse. Top off dinner with a plate of anise biscotti and a dish of leather and silk (licorice and chocolate chip) ice cream. After

Licorice at the Bar
("objection!" "overruLed.")

One of the most common places to find licorice-flavored products is in the liquor cabinet. There are several licorice-flavored liqueurs and dozens of ways to enjoy them. Licorice-flavored liqueurs are commonly served after dinner as an evening cordial to aid digestion. The most common are:

Pernod: This French anise-based, yellowish liqueur is a key ingredient in bouillabaisse, the famous French fish stew, and Sazerac, a well-known New Orleans cocktail. Very popular in France, Pernod is usually mixed with water, which turns it whitish and cloudy.

Pastis: This licorice-flavored cordial, popular in the south of France, contains fewer ingredients than Pernod and is therefore not as complex. Like Pernod, pastis is usually mixed with water, which turns it whitish and cloudy. Pastis is the heir of the infamous absinthe, a potent, bitter liqueur (reputedly first brewed by witches) distilled from the bitter-tasting shrub wormwood (which contains a mild hallucinogen and was used in the middle ages to counteract spells designed to hinder sexual potency) and flavored with a variety of herbs including anise. Absinthe was banned in the early part of the twentieth century because it was often abused, and caused dangerous side effects such as convulsions, hallucinations, and even death. (Sort of like an Agent Orange cocktail.) However, there has been a revival recently, and it still can be purchased in England and a few Eastern European countries with really bad economies.

Anisette: This licorice-flavored liqueur made with anise seed is very sweet and is used in many mixed drinks.

Pacharan: This pink, sweet liqueur is made from anisette and pacharan, or sloe berries. Its origins date back many centuries to the distilled products made by wine growers in Navarra, a province in northern Spain. It can be enjoyed, like other anise-flavored beverages, as an aperitif, an after-dinner drink, or an ingredient in light cocktails.

Ouzo: This strong, slightly sweet, fragrant, anise-flavored Greek spirit is usually diluted with two parts water for each part ouzo, which turns it whitish and opaque. It is a great accompaniment to the strong-flavored, cured fish and cheeses of the Greek islands.

Sambuca: This liqueur is made by an infusion of witch elder bush and licorice. Often flavored with sweet anise, it is similar to anisette but has a higher alcoholic content, a slight coffee flavor, and is not as sweet. Sambuca is a key ingredient in hundreds of cocktails (the kind you drank in college, resulting in a guaranteed hangover) ranging from an AK-47 (apple schnapps, rum, tequila, Tia Maria, and Sambuca) to a Zebra (Sambuca and tequila).

Jägermeister: This bitter German licorice liqueur is made from a complex blend of 56 herbs, fruits, and spices. It should be served cold to tame its assertive herbal flavor, which resembles cough syrup. Jägermeister, which means "hunt master" in German, is useful in concocting dozens of obscure cocktails such as The Little Green Man from Mars (Jägermeister and Rumpleminze garnished with a mint-green maraschino cherry, without stem. Just perfect for Saint Patrick's Day puking), and Sex with an Alligator (Jägermeister, melon liqueur, raspberry liqueur, pineapple juice, and ice), a very cute cocktail for girls who like drinks with silly names and partners whose names they can't remember.

you've discovered the power that licorice can have on the affection connection, you'll be a licorice lover for life.

Remember, once you go black there's no turning back.

The Cooking Couple's Licorice Menu for Amour

Here are a few of our favorite quick and easy ways to ignite romance with licorice and its kissing cousins.

For a licorice-inspired cocktail hour, try one of these drinks.

{ Black Licorice }

1¼ ounce Sambuca
½ ounce coconut liqueur
2 ounces light cream
Blend Sambuca, coconut liqueur, and light cream with 1 cup ice until smooth. Serve in a parfait glass garnished with a black licorice stick.

{ Jelly Bean Shooter }

1 ounce anisette
1 ounce blackberry brandy
Layer anisette and blackberry brandy in a shot glass, or serve on the rocks.

{ Sazerac }

½ teaspoon Pernod or other absinthe substitute (Use real absinthe if you can get it, but don't complain to us about dead brain cells and your nightlong conversation with Jim Morrison.)
Dash Peychaud's bitters
½ teaspoon simple syrup
2 ounces whiskey
Coat a chilled old-fashioned glass by pouring in Pernod and swirling the glass. Add the simple syrup and bitters. Fill with whiskey and garnish with a twist.

{ Fennel Salad }

Serve with French bread and freshly grated Parmesan cheese, and you have an easy, elegant side dish or first course that's light and just right for an aphrodisiac-inspired meal.
1 medium fennel bulb, thinly sliced

4 spring or canned artichokes, cooked and halved

¾ cup lemon juice

½ cup extra virgin olive oil

Salt and pepper to taste

Toss sliced fennel with artichokes, lemon juice, and olive oil. Let marinate for about 30 minutes and serve.

{ creamy fennel soup with shrimp }

Fennel soup is still enjoyed in parts of the Mediterranean as an aphrodisiac. Onions, garlic, Pernod, and shrimp add to the recipe's appeal as Cupid cuisine.

2 tablespoons butter

1 pound fresh fennel (about 1 large bulb) with greens

1 onion, peeled and chopped

2 cloves garlic, chopped

3 cups chicken stock

⅔ cup light cream

1 tablespoon Pernod

Salt and freshly ground pepper to taste

½ pound small cooked shrimp, peeled and deveined

1. Clean and chop the fennel bulb, reserving any greens for garnish.
2. In a large soup pot, melt the butter over medium-low heat. Sauté the fennel and onion until soft, 5 to 6 minutes. Add the garlic and sauté for another 1 to 2 minutes.
3. Pour in the chicken stock and simmer until the fennel is very tender. Purée the mixture in a food processor or blender until smooth.
4. Pour the soup back in the pot, and add the cream and Pernod. Bring to a simmer and add salt and pepper to taste.
5. To serve, place several shrimp (about 6) in each bowl. Ladle soup around shrimp and garnish with reserved fennel greens.

Serves 4

{ sweet & savory Bouillabaisse }

The inclusion of several types of shellfish gives this dish an extra
aphrodisiacal kick. It's also quick, easy, delicious, and light.

1 tablespoon olive oil

1 medium onion, diced

½ teaspoon fennel seeds

1 cup canned tomatoes with their juice

½ teaspoon orange zest

1 cup dry white wine

1 cup clam broth

½ teaspoon fresh tarragon leaves or ⅛ teaspoon dried tarragon

Pinch of saffron

1 clove garlic, split, plus 2 teaspoons minced

12 clams or mussels, scrubbed and washed

¾ pound white-fleshed fish fillets (such as cod, halibut, or sea bass)
    cut into chunks

¾ pound shellfish (preferably a mixture of shrimp and scallops)

1 tablespoon anise-flavored liqueur such as Pernod

Salt and freshly ground black pepper to taste

6 slices ½-inch-thick crusty French bread, toasted

2 tablespoons minced fresh parsley

1. In a large soup kettle, heat oil. Add onions and cook over medium
   heat until soft, about 7 minutes.

2. Add fennel, tomatoes, orange zest, wine, broth, tarragon, saffron,
   and minced garlic. Bring to a boil, cover, and simmer for 10 minutes. Rub toast with split garlic and set aside.

3. Add clams or mussels and simmer, covered, for about 5 minutes.
   Add the fish chunks and cook for an additional 5 minutes. When the
   mussels or clams open, add shellfish and anise-flavored liqueur.
   Cover and cook until shellfish are cooked through, approximately
   5 minutes. Taste and adjust seasoning.

4. To serve, place two pieces toasted French bread in bottom of a
   soup bowl. Ladle fish and broth over the bread, sprinkle with parsley, and enjoy.

Generously serves 2

{ Leather and silk ice cream }
(Licorice chocolate chip ice cream)

The combination of licorice and chocolate may seem a little odd, but they work beautifully together, both on the libido and the taste buds.

1½ cups whole milk

1½ cups heavy cream

⅔ cup sugar

1 large egg plus 2 egg yolks

2 tablespoons Pernod or anisette liqueur

1 teaspoon vanilla extract

½ cup chocolate chips

1. In a heavy saucepan combine the milk, cream, and ⅓ cup sugar. Cook over medium-high heat, stirring occasionally, until mixture reaches 175° F.
2. Combine egg, egg yolks, and remaining sugar and whisk with an electric mixer or by hand until thick and pale yellow.
3. Slowly add ½ cup of the milk/cream mixture to the egg mixture, whisking vigorously. Whisk mixture back into the saucepan and cook over low heat until mixture reaches 180° F. Stir in Pernod or anisette and vanilla extract.
4. Cool mixture completely, stir, and place in ice cream machine. Freeze according to manufacturer's instructions. Stir in chocolate chips and chill in freezer.

If you don't have an ice cream machine or don't have the time to make ice cream from scratch, simply soften 1 quart vanilla ice cream. Stir in 2 tablespoons Pernod or anisette, along with ½ cup chocolate chips. Refreeze and enjoy. Personally, when the licorice takes effect we can think of much better things to do than churning ice cream.

Makes about 1 quart

{ Licorice Biscotti }

1 cup sugar
½ cup butter (1 stick), softened
1 teaspoon licorice or anise extract
2 eggs
3½ cups flour
1 teaspoon baking powder
½ teaspoon salt
¾ cup almonds (whole, slivered, or sliced)

1. Heat oven to 350° F. In a large bowl, beat sugar, butter, licorice or anise extract, and eggs using an electric mixer on medium speed until light, fluffy, and lemon-colored. Stir in flour, baking powder, salt, and almonds. Mix by hand until a dough forms.
2. Divide dough in half. Shape each half into a 10x3-inch rectangle. Place on ungreased cookie sheet. Bake about 20 minutes, until toothpick inserted into the center of the dough comes out clean. Let dough cool for 15 minutes.
3. Cut into ½-inch slices. Turn slices on their side and place on cookie sheet. Bake until light brown and crisp, about 15 minutes. Let cool on a wire rack.

Makes 3 to 4 dozen cookies

6

Juicy Fruits

I always determine the sexual capabilities of a woman by the way she eats fruit.

—Gabriele D'Annunzio, Italian poet, novelist, and soldier who lived from 1863 to 1938

Fruit was the first seduction food. In the Biblical account of the fall of man, the serpent enticed Eve with an unspecified forbidden fruit growing in the middle of the Garden of Eden. Eve found the fruit good to eat, a delight to the eyes, and desirable as a source of wisdom, so she took a bite and gave the fruit to Adam, who also ate.

Well, you know the rest of the story. When God caught wind of what they had done, their eternal Paradise membership card was revoked. If Eve hadn't eaten the forbidden fruit we'd still be hanging out naked in Paradise having a grand old time.

You first parents of the human race . . . who ruined yourself for an apple, what might you have done for a truffled turkey?

—Brillat-Savarin

Because it is naturally sweet and delectable, bears the seeds that create life, and grows above the earth toward heaven, people have always celebrated fruit, used it as an aphrodisiac, and offered it to their deities.

Both figs and grapes were associated with Dionysus, the god of wine, fertility, and procreation. Ancient Jews used fruit as part of their courtship ritual. Pomegranates, which are impregnated with hundreds of seeds covered in sweet-tart fruit, were eaten at Babylonian wedding feasts. The Chinese considered peaches and apricots to be erotic, sensual symbols for ripe sexuality. Melon soup is also eaten to stimulate the libido. In Europe a favorite love casserole was made from steamed dates and ham. And prunes, which are believed to be sexually stimulating, were given free of charge to clients in Elizabethan brothels.

One of nature's healthiest foods, fruit is ideal for fueling both sexual and overall vitality. Easy to digest, full of complex carbohydrates (an excellent energy source), water, and important vitamins and minerals, high in fiber, and almost always low in fat and calories, fruit is the perfect antidote for commonly consumed, overprocessed, sweet snacks and desserts. Fruits come in a wide variety of shapes, colors, and flavors. They are portable, sweet, and crunchy, too.

Eating perfectly ripe fruit is a transcendently voluptuous experience. Sensual, sweet, juicy, naked, raw, and delicious, ready to offer its passion without pretension or preparation to the gods of romance, love, and lust; fruit is mankind's first aphrodisiac. Was

what is a fruit?

Botanically, a fruit is defined as the dry or fleshy developed ovary of a plant that surrounds a seed or seeds. Or the edible part of a plant produced from a flower. Most of us think of fruit as sweet, juicy produce that grows on a plant or a tree. However you define it, fruit's life mission is to spread seeds.

By contrast, vegetables are herbaceous (nonwoody, green, and leafy) plants grown for their edible parts (roots, leaves, stems, or flowers). Vegetables are usually blander than fruits and are eaten as part of the main course instead of dessert.

it worth getting thrown out of Paradise for? Take a bite and you decide.

Nature's dessert also has a secret attribute. In the words of Italian poet and author Gabriele D'Annunzio, fruit reveals whether a lover is good in bed. According to D'Annunzio, "Small, mincing bites—the ladylike kind—are not good. But if she crunches the fruit, salivates with pleasure, and crinkles her nose in enjoyment, this girl, my friend, should prove to be a redoubtable love partner."

For a vivid portrait of the seductive power of fruit, watch what Nastassja Kinski does to a strawberry in Roman Polanski's *Tess*. Or look at Edouard Manet's scandalous painting *Dejeuner sur l'Herbe*, "Luncheon on the Grass." (It hangs in the Musee d'Orsay in Paris, but you can easily see a good reproduction on the Internet or in an art history book.) After you check out the nude woman sitting next to the two clothed men, take a look at the seductive picnic in the lower left-hand corner of the painting. The basket is overflowing with juicy, ripe fruits, obviously placed there by the artist as a symbol of the sexual nature of the subject.

How about creating your own "Luncheon on the Grass" and putting fruit to your personal aphrodisiac test. To get you started, here is a list of some of our favorite juicy fruits.

A IS For AppLe

Like an apple tree among the trees of the forest, so is my beloved among the young men.

—song of solomon 2:3

Although the apple was not the forbidden fruit that got Adam and Eve kicked out of Paradise (more on this later), this popular fruit has a long history as an aphrodisiac and symbol for love and sex.

The seventeenth-century English naturalist, philosopher, and theologian John Ray wrote, "An apple, an egg, and a nut, you may eat after a slut."

The *Ancren Riwle,* a thirteenth-century guidebook for English nuns, describes apples as "a token of everything that arouses lust and sensual delights."

In Greek mythology, Aphrodite won the golden apple of discord when Paris (the man who later abducted Helen of Troy, triggering the Trojan War), judged her as the most beautiful goddess. The Greeks and Romans found the apple erotic, and lovers commonly threw apples at each other (ouch!) and exchanged them as gifts.

In the Bible the author of the Song of Solomon writes: "Refresh me with apples, because I am lovesick."

Apples have been used as euphemisms for testicles and breasts, and an "apple monger" is slang for a pimp. Today we describe people we love as "the apple of my eye."

During the Middle Ages in Germany women soaked apples in their perspiration and gave them to their lovers to increase passion. We're not sure how they collected the required sweat, but as outlandish as this trick sounds, it was probably a very effective way to transmit pheromones.

People who practice the faith of the Yoruba tribe in Africa and Santeria offer apples to a deity called Chango, the thunder god who rules over male fertility.

Hindus make a love potion from white thorn apples, black pepper, honey, and long pepper. We don't recommend trying this one at home. Thorn apples (jimsonweed or *Datura stramonium*) contain chemicals similar to mandrake, another well-known, dangerous aphrodisiac, and are extremely toxic.

One of the first cultivated fruits (its ancestor was a small, sour fruit similar to a crabapple), apples, in both fresh and dried form, have been eaten since ancient times. Today the average American eats nearly twenty pounds of apples a year. There are between 7,000 and 8,000 varieties of apples, but only a small fraction (around 100) are grown commercially in the United States. Red Delicious, Golden Delicious, Granny Smith, Macin-

An Apple a Day

An apple a day can indeed help keep the doctor, as well as the dentist, away. They are rich in the disease-fighting phytochemical quercetin, and a great source of both soluble and insoluble fiber, which can help keep cholesterol levels low. Apples also help cleanse the teeth and contain a multitude of vitamins and minerals. All for under a hundred calories!

tosh, Rome Beauty, Jonathan, York, and Stayman are among the most popular types and make up 80 percent of the American apple harvest.

Although apples store well they taste best when fresh—especially with a wedge of American cheddar. Look for apples that are firm, not mushy, and store them in the refrigerator.

To use apples as a love food, we recommend adding aphrodisiacal nuts and spices such as cinnamon, nutmeg, or ginger to various apple-based dishes: apple pie, baked apples, and apple crisp. You can also cook apples with meat dishes or incorporate them into stuffings and fruit salad. Of course, you can always just emulate Eve: take a bite and grab a fig leaf.

R is for Avocado

One of the most rare and pleasant fruits of the island. It nourisheth and strengtheneth the body.

—W. Hughes, British royal physician,
describing the avocado

The name for this R-rated fruit comes from the Aztec word for testicle, *ahucatl*. Avocados are shaped like testicles, hang in pairs like testicles, and, well . . . you get the idea. The Aztecs made a sexually potent spread from mashed avocados, chiles, onions, and tomatoes called *ahuaca-mull.* Today, we call it guacamole. Like the ancient Aztecs, modern Mexicans still eat avocados as an aphrodisiac.

From the tables of Cortez (where the fruit was frequently eaten with salt and pepper or sugar, and the seeds were used to make indelible ink), the avocado traveled to the decadent kingdoms of Europe. The Sun King (Louis XIV) nicknamed avocados *la bonne poire* (the good pear) because he believed they restored his lagging libido.

The British living in Jamaica called the fruit "alligator-pear," perhaps because the skin of an avocado resembles that of an alligator; and English sailors referred to avocados as midshipman's butter after they learned to use the fruit as a tasty spread that improved their sea rations. Because of its stimulating reputation, Catholic priests dubbed it a forbidden fruit and told their congregants not to eat it.

Film star Mae West was perhaps the twentieth century's most influential avocado aphrodisiac advocate. She was said to eat at least one per day, and to attribute her robust sexual appetite and well-preserved looks to this rich fruit.

The three original types of avocados—Mexican, Guatemalan, and West Indian—have been cultivated for about 7,000 years. Today, avocados are also grown in America (in both Florida and California), Africa, and Australia.

Avocados do not ripen until after they are picked because avocado tree leaves produce a hormone that inhibits the fruit-ripening chemical ethylene. To tell if an avocado is ripe, squeeze it gently. Ripe fruit, which can be stored in the refrigerator for 4 to 5 days, will be firm yet yield to gentle pressure. You can speed up the ripening process by placing the fruit in a paper bag for several days. (Add a banana if you are really in a hurry. Bananas contain an abundance of ethylene, a plant hormone that accelerates ripening.)

Avocados and Health

Avocados are one of the few fruits that are high in fat. (Most of it is the heart-healthy monounsaturated kind.) They are also the fruit richest in protein, vitamin E, and beta carotene. The average avocado contains about 30 grams of fat and 4 to 5 grams of protein, and weighs in at about 300 calories. Avocados are also rich in the cholesterol-lowering compound beta-sitosterol and the antioxidant glutathione.

Mashed avocados can be applied to the hair for 5 minutes to add luster, or mixed with honey and lime juice and used as a moisturizing mask. If used as a hair treatment, we do not recommend recycling for aphrodisiacal use.

Avocados can become bitter when heated, and so are best eaten raw. Once your avocado is ripe, cut it in half with a knife, pry out the pit, and scoop out the flesh. Mashed avocado makes a wonderful sandwich spread with fewer calories and fat than butter, mayonnaise, margarine, or cream cheese. You can also use diced avocado as a garnish, omelet filling, burger topping, or an addition to salads. Halved avocados make a handy edible cup for seafood salads, and the puréed fruit makes a delicious cold soup.

The Banana: The Breakfast of Champions

Eat the banana;
I look at him;
I give him the banana
As the banana is with me now,
So will the man be with me

—Irish Love Chant

Because of their erotic appearance as well as their sweet, rich, creamy taste, bananas have been considered an aphrodisiac since people first tasted the fruit in Southeast Asia thousands of years ago. The butt of many jokes (in early-twentieth-century Britain, "I had a banana with Lady Diana" meant you had just had sex), and used often as a body double for health educators demonstrating how to use condoms, the word *banana* is still frequently used as slang for "penis." In Hawaii, because of their shape, bananas were once *kapu,* off-limits to women.

Many cultures, including Islam, believed the banana was the forbidden fruit eaten by Adam and Eve in the Garden of Eden. (A banana peel was probably more effective in covering Adam's appendage than a fig leaf.) In India, bananas are offered to Hindu gods, and the leaves adorn marriage altars.

Bananas also have an intellectual side. Their scientific name is *Musa sapitum,* meaning "fruit of the wise men." According to Indian legend, bananas were a favorite food of sages, who also liked to rest under the shade of banana plants.

Bananas actually don't grow on trees. The banana plant belongs to the genus *Musa* (which also includes other aphrodisiacs like ginger and lilies), and is the world's biggest herb. The fruit of the banana plant is actually considered a berry.

Nutritionally speaking, the average medium-sized banana contains about one hundred calories and is a good source of fiber, potassium, and tryptophan, an amino acid that promotes relaxation. According to a recent Harvard study, eating just two potas-

Banana Buzz

During the sixties, banana peels, which contain small amounts of the neurotransmitters serotonin, dopamine, and norepinephrine, were smoked as a replacement for marijuana. However, smoking peels didn't get people high, and the fad quickly peeled out.

sium-rich bananas a day can have a major impact on lowering high blood pressure. The easy-to-digest fruit is frequently recommended as a first food for patients recovering from illness of the gastrointestinal tract.

Until two businessmen began importing the fruit in large numbers from the Caribbean, bananas were a pricey luxury. Today, bananas and plantains (often called cooking bananas), are the fourth largest fruit crop in the world, affordable and widely cultivated across the tropics. There are many types of bananas, from the sharp-tasting silk banana to the tiny baby or nino variety. Most of the bananas we eat are Cavendish.

Bananas can be used to make smoothies, sweets such as the spiced Indian dish panchamrutham, fritters, and of course banana bread and muffins. When cooking with bananas, make sure the fruit is at the right stage of ripeness—yellow in color, with no green and a minimum of brown spots. Ripe bananas can also be frozen and eaten, or saved for later use in recipes.

The Fertile Fig

If I should wish a fruit brought to Paradise it would certainly be the fig.

—Muhammad

Like bananas, figs are exhibitionists. Long considered phallic and an aphrodisiac, the fruit was a Hindu symbol for the Lingam (penis) and Yoni (vagina). At one time the fig leaf, which resembles a penis and a pair of testicles, was believed to have the same sexually stimulating powers as the herb mandrake.

On the outside, a whole fresh fig resembles a penis. Cut in half, the inside looks like female genitals. Now take a bite, let the fruit seduce you, and you'll quickly realize why figs, which are indigenous to Persia, Syria, and Asia Minor, have been savored since prehistoric times and celebrated for centuries.

The fig is the most frequently mentioned fruit in the Bible, and pictures of figs are depicted on Egyptian tombs. The fruit was used to honor Thoth, the god of wisdom, and the sun god, Amon-Ra. Cleopatra adored figs and practically died eating them. (The asp that killed her lay in a basket of figs.)

The ancient Greeks, who linked the sacred fruit with fertility and love, held fig orgies honoring Dionysus and the fig harvest by dropping their fig leaves and having ritualistic sex. For a flavor of those celebrations, consider these lines from the Greek dramatist Aristophanes:

Now live splendidly together,
Free from adversity
Pick figs
May his be large and hard,
May hers be sweet

Ancient Athenians ate the fruit daily and called themselves *philosykos,* literally, "friends of the fig." Figs were so important and special that Solon, the ruler of Attica from 639 to 559 B.C., made exporting figs illegal. The Romans celebrated New Year's by exchanging figs, linked the fruit with Bacchus (their god of wine) and Saturn (their god of the harvest), and used them in love potions. According to the Roman poet Horace, one such tasty potion was made from "wild figs growing on a grave," "bones snatched from the mouth of a hungry bitch," and "feathers of a screech owl." That's one we don't suggest trying at home.

However, if you're planning a wedding you may want to have guests incorporate the Southern European custom of throwing figs (instead of rice) at the bride and groom to encourage a fertile union. Whether you're hitched or not, we recommend following the lead of the Greeks and celebrating the first figs of summer by feeding each other ripe figs and having sex.

Though the fruit is sacred to many cultures, the word *fig* has also been used as sexual slang in others. "Nibbling a fig" is an

Fig Nutrition

Figs are restorative. They increase the strength of young people, preserve the elderly in better health, and make them look younger with fewer wrinkles.

—Pliny the Elder, Roman writer

The first fitness fruit, figs were eaten by ancient Olympic athletes as a training food to increase strength and speed, and Olympic champions were presented with fig laurels.

In the Bible, Hezekiah, king of Judah, used figs as a remedy for boils. Interestingly, psoralens, a chemical in figs, promotes tanning, and is one remedy for skin pigmentation diseases.

When it comes to fiber and mineral content figs lead the fruit pack. One serving (about 1½ dried figs) contains one-fifth of the daily value for fiber, 244 mg of potassium, 53 mg of calcium, and 1.2 mg of iron, all for only 60 calories.

Arabic term for cunnilingus, and "fig you" is the auditory equivalent of giving someone the finger.

Botanically, the fig is actually not a fruit, but a cluster of nearly 1,500 minuscule flowers that lie inside the fig and turn into tiny fruits called drupes that resemble seeds. Each fig contains both male and female flowers that can't fertilize each other, because the female flower is ready to be impregnated before the male flower makes pollen. (Kind of like the reverse of premature ejaculation.) The fig relies on a tiny insect called a fig wasp that crawls inside the fig for the winter and emerges in the spring covered with pollen, ready to impregnate a different fertile fig.

There are hundreds of varieties of figs, but only a few are grown and eaten in America. All dried figs cultivated in the U.S. come from California, where over 30 million pounds a year are harvested at the end of the summer and beginning of the fall. The most common figs grown in this country are:

- *The Mission Fig* (also called Common or Franciscana). Named for Spanish missionaries who planted fig trees as they traveled north through California, this flavorful, sweet fig is deep purple on the outside and reddish-brown inside.
- *The Kadota Fig.* An Italian transplant known as Dattato, this thick-skinned yellow-green fig with an amber interior is available fresh, dried, and canned.
- *The Calimyrna Fig.* This large, amber, slightly nutty fruit resembles the first figs that were grown in Asia Minor 2,000 years ago. Known as Smyrna in Turkey and Greece, they were brought to California in 1882 and renamed for their new home.
- *The Adriatic Fig.* Imported from the Mediterranean, this fig is very sweet, dries well, and is often used to make fig bars.

A perfectly ripe fig is a sweet treat that everyone should experience. Beneath the soft, velvety skin lies succulent, buttery flesh that oozes sweetness and sensuality.

who the heck was newton?

The famous Fig Newton made its first appearance in 1892, and was invented by James Hazen, bakery manager for the New York Biscuit Company. The cookies were named after Newton, a Boston suburb, because Hazen had already named a number of cookies in his line (Beacon Hill, Melrose, and Brighton) after other Boston suburbs. "What, no Red Sox cookie?" "Maybe when they finally win something they'll get a cookie named after them."

Fresh figs, which are highly perishable and should be enjoyed as soon as they ripen, work beautifully in both sweet and savory dishes. As an appetizer, halved figs pair well with thinly sliced proscuitto and can also be wrapped in bacon, broiled for about 10 minutes, and served alone or as part of a salad. Mild soft cheeses (such as chèvre, mascarpone, and ricotta) and figs complement each other nicely. For a decadent dessert, whole figs can be baked in butter, or poached in port or orange juice with a dash of fruit-flavored liqueur and topped with cream. Sliced fresh figs also make a nice addition to fruit tarts and fruit salads.

Chopped dried figs, which have a long shelf life, can be added to muffins, cookies, and breads; stirred into oatmeal, grain dishes, stuffings, and salsas; or combined with olive oil and rosemary for a pizza or focaccia topping. The dried fruit can also be puréed and used to sweeten and flavor yogurt, ice cream, or baked goods.

The Grapes of Romance

Wine has . . . inspired invention, animated religion, made men vociferous, nourished beliefs, kindled wrath, provoked love and lust, and softened hard beds.

–The London Times, "wine merchants uncorked"

The party animal of the plant kingdom, grapes and their fermented juice, wine, have been enjoyed and celebrated since at least Neolithic times (8500 to 4000 B.C.). Wine, the drink of romance, was first produced around 6000 B.C. in Mesopotamia and Caucassia, and since then has had a major impact on world civilization and romance. In poetry, prose, and in bed, from antiquity to modern times, from candle-lit dinners to drunken orgies, wine has always been glorified as a sexual stimulant.

Dionysus (known as Bacchus by the Romans, hence the term "bacchanalia") was the god of wine, fertility, and procreation (funny how those three things go together). This is why bunches of grapes were given to newlyweds to insure fertility. In the words of Ambrose Bierce, "He [Bacchus] was a convenient deity, invented by the ancients as an excuse for getting drunk." In honor of the god, the Romans frequently drank wine and held naked orgies in wine-filled public baths.

The Romans loved grapes and wine so much that they planted grapes, which are native to the area bordered by the Black and Caspian Seas and Afghanistan, throughout their empire. Noah, who needed all the help he could get to repopulate the earth, planted a vineyard almost immediately after he came out of the ark.

One of the most luscious and suggestive of fruits, grapes are used throughout romantic literature to describe women. In the Bible's Song of Solomon, the fruit is compared to a woman's breasts, and the Roman poet Catullus describes a young woman as being so seductive that she should "be hid like ripe black grapes." The sex symbol Mae West is famous for her provocative line from the movie *She Done Him Wrong:* "Beulah, peel me a grape!"

Grapes are a great place for you and your beloved to begin your exploration of aphrodisiacal fruit. Feed each other the juicy fruit. Press your lips together and share a solitary orb. Or simply open a nice bottle of Chardonnay or Burgundy and toast your love. Sharing a bottle of wine stimulates the libido and turns an ordinary meal into an erotic encounter.

Where there is no wine there is no love.

–Euripides, Greek dramatist

Wine, food, and love—the three Musketeers of romance—were made for each other, which is why they are linked throughout literature.

•The Roman comic playwright Terence wrote, "*Sine Ceres et Libero friget Venus*" "Without Ceres (the mother goddess associated with food) and Libero (Bacchus, the god of wine), Venus (the goddess of love) will freeze." Venus was rarely frigid. According to Greek legend she and Bacchus made love on at least one occa-

The French Paradox

*Wine is at the head of all medicines; where wine is lack-
ing, drugs are necessary.*

–Babylonian Talmud: Baba Bathra

In France, artery-clogging foods like full-fat cheese, butter, foie
gras, and cream flow like the Seine, yet rates of heart disease are
much lower in France than they are in America. The phenomenon is
called the French Paradox, and scientists think that moderate consumption of wine, especially red, is responsible for the 25 to 40
percent lower rate of heart disease in France despite the high consumption of fat and cholesterol.

There are a number of reasons wine is so good for you and your
heart. First, a number of studies have found that the alcohol in wine,
beer, and spirits prevents the development of atherosclerosis (hard-
ening of the arteries) by increasing levels of HDL, the good cholesterol that transports bad cholesterol away from the arteries to the
liver where it can be disposed of. Second, chemicals (resveratrol,
catechin, quercetin, and epicatechin) found in grape skin remain in
red wine and are strong antioxidants, which can protect you from
heart disease and may also help prevent cancer. Third, like aspirin,
wine helps prevent blood clots that can lead to heart attacks and
strokes.

Unlike spirits, which numb the taste buds, wine has many flavor
components and complements food. It whets the appetite and is a
wonderful accompaniment to a romantic meal and evening. Wine can
also kill bacteria, so drinking it with dinner may help prevent or
lessen the effects of food poisoning. The wines most often mentioned
as aphrodisiacs include champagne (Casanova's favorite), claret,
Chablis, Chianti, Sauternes, and Burgundy. When describing a seductive meal, the Marquis de Sade recommended Burgundy, claret,
champagne, Hermitage, tokyo (an exceptional wine from Hungary),
Madeira, and Falernia.

sion and the result was Priapus, the phallic god of fertility. Another reason why wine and love are a classic combination.

·Omar Khayyám, the eleventh- and twelfth-century Persian mathematician, philosopher, and astronomer, is famous for his line from *The Rubaiyat,* "A loaf of bread, a jug of wine, and thou."

·The German poet Johann Wolfgang von Goethe, when asked which three things he would bring to an island, said, "Poetry [his food], a beautiful woman, and enough bottles of the world's finest wines to survive this dry period!"

Wine has the ability to transform our state of mind so that we are more in the mood for love. In the *Art of Love,* Ovid, the popular Roman poet, commented, "When there is plenty of wine, sorrow and worry take wing."

W. B. Yeats summed it up best when he wrote:

Wine comes in at the mouth
And love comes in at the eye;
That's all we shall know for truth
Before we grow old and die.
I lift the glass to my mouth,
I look at you, and I sigh.

Studies have found that for men, simply expecting that they are going to drink can increase sexual arousal and decrease inhibition. Small amounts of alcohol also can increase levels of dopamine, a key neurotransmitter for a healthy sexual response. According to a study published in the British journal *Nature,* alcohol may also increase levels of testosterone, the hormone responsible for libido in both sexes, in women. However, studies show excessive consumption of alcohol in men quickly decreases testosterone levels and impairs sexual performance. Moderate consumption of alcohol can also help improve blood circulation, and as you will learn in Chapter 10, "The Cooking Couple's Best Sex Diet," healthy circulation means pumped-up genitals, which is one key to a healthy sex life.

wine basics

Wine is a living, breathing food and so must be stored correctly unless you want to drink a beverage that resembles vinegar more than Chardonnay. Here are a few tips to keep in mind.

•Store wine in a dark place (exposure to sunlight turns wine brown) at a low, consistent temperature. Between 50° F and 60° F is ideal.

•To prevent oxygen from entering the wine and to keep corks from drying out, store bottles horizontally.

•Do not disturb. Agitating wine can shake up sediment and alter the way the wine ages.

•To keep corks moist and labels from falling, humidity should be between 70 and 75 percent.

coffee is for lovers

Coffee should be black as Hell, strong as death, and sweet as love.

–Turkish proverb

America's favorite morning drink, coffee, is an aphrodisiac as well as a fruit. The most popular beverage in the world, coffee's annual global consumption is about 400 billion cups. Coffee drinkers report having sex more frequently and enjoying it more than non-coffee drinkers. And while we may take that first cup of joe for granted, according to Turkish law, not providing your wife with coffee was once grounds for divorce.

Coffee works as a sexual stimulant on several levels. Small amounts of caffeine can help excite the mind and energize the body, both of which can put you in the mood for sex. Studies also show that coffee can increase levels of dopamine, that neurotransmitter needed for a healthy libido and sex life. And caffeine

Tea for two

If your partner is a tea lover, never fear. The breakfast beverage is also considered to be an aphrodisiac in the Orient. Prostitutes in Asian countries make a potent syrup from two ounces of tea simmered in a gallon of water for 24 hours. The syrup is mixed with sweetened water and served to clients.

Gunpowder tea, a green tea from China, is thought to be a particularly effective aphrodisiac. Its namesake, gunpowder, was actually consumed by America's first cowboys as an aphrodisiac. (This is another one we don't recommend trying at home.) The cowboys mixed a teaspoon of black gunpowder with a shot of rum in a large mug of hot water. The aphro buzz came from the combination of alcohol, which boosted the libido, and gunpowder, which irritated the urinary tract. Our question: out on the trail, what were they going to have sex with? "Move along, little dogie."

gives both circulation and metabolism a boost, helping blood flow to the genitals.

So the next time your lover says he or she is not in the mood, prepare them a fresh cup of java with just the right balance of sugar and cream. If you really want to make the boudoir boil, present the steaming cup on a tray with a rose and a wonderful piece of chocolate, and enjoy a cup of coffee together in bed for a little morning amour.

Coffee is actually a form of fruit juice that is generally made by brewing dried, roasted, and ground coffee beans (which are actually berries, called coffee cherries) with water. According to legend, the berries were first discovered by an Arab shepherd who observed that his goats became rather perky after munching on coffee cherries.

Initially, coffee cherries were eaten whole or with fat. Next they were mashed, allowed to ferment, and made into a type of wine. Around A.D. 1000 people started drying the fruit, and by A.D. 1300 the dried beans were roasted and made into a beverage called *Qahwah* (a poetic name for wine), used in religious rituals (you could pray all night long) as a substitute for wine.

Merchants from Venice brought coffee from Arabia to Europe in 1615. Coffee's caffeine kick and exotic allure quickly caught on throughout Western Europe. By the middle of the eighteenth century, the beverage was popular in cafés in London, among the elite of Paris, and with artists like Balzac, Voltaire, and Bach.

Initially, Arabic merchants tried to maintain a coffee monopoly by making it illegal to export fertile beans. The tight control was broken by an Indian man named Baba Budan, who strapped seven seeds to his body and smuggled them out of Arabia. Today coffee grows in warm climates throughout the world and is the second largest world commodity after oil.

Napoléon Nightcap

Way before Starbucks, double mochas, and frappaccinos, Josephine purportedly invented a coffee beverage that contained two other aphrodisiacs, chocolate and lavender, and served it as an aphrodisiac to her husband, Napoléon. Make it at home and see if it works for your little Bonaparte.

2 tablespoons freshly ground coffee beans

¼ cup fresh English lavender* flowers (This type of lavender, *Lavendula angustifolia,* is the only type suitable for cooking.)

1 cup hot chocolate

Place the coffee beans and lavender in a glass bowl. Add 1 cup boiling water. Let mixture steep for 2 to 3 minutes, and pour through a strainer. Mix with the hot chocolate. Pour into mugs and enjoy.

*Lavender has been used in love potions since at least the Middle Ages. Shakespeare wrote in The Winter's Tale that hot lavender is very stimulating when "given to men of middle age."

other Erotic Fruits

Strawberries. Dipped in chocolate or whipped cream, combined with champagne (a classic aphrodisiac), or slowly nibbled naked, strawberries (aka fruit nipples for you lovers of erotic literature) are an extremely sensual, suggestive, and sexy fruit. Just feed each other the fruit or lick strawberry juice off your lover's lips and you'll see what we mean. The fruit also has a legacy of magic and mystery. Strawberries were a forbidden fruit to early Greeks, who banned all red foods from the diet, and pregnant women in medieval times avoided the berry because they believed eating it would cause the child to be born with a strawberry birthmark.

There is nothing more deliciously sensual than a strawberry dipped in melted chocolate. Strawberries are to chocolate what bread is to peanut butter. The perfect pedestal.

Durian. There is a Malaysian saying, "When the durians come down, the sarongs come off." This large, green, spiky fruit (a native of Southeast Asia, where it is called "the king of fruit") has quite the reputation as an aphrodisiac. Whether it's due to chemicals in the fruit or its unique heady aroma (which has been described as a combination of compost, garlic, and rancid cheese), custard-like texture, and intense flavor, durian puts people in the mood for love. Just don't eat it on Singapore's mass transit system, where it has been banned. (Are they worried about a rush-hour orgy?) Durian is extremely hard to find in America. The best place to look is in Asian produce markets in May, when the fruit is in season.

Papaya. More accessible than durian, this tropical fruit, with its small, shiny black seeds and sweet perfumy flesh, contains an enzyme called papian that can help you digest all those other aphrodisiacs in your love banquet. In Cuba, the fruit is referred to as a *fruta bomba* (bomb fruit) because the word *papaya* is slang for the female genitals.

Mango. Also known as the king of fruit, and described as "sealed jars of paradisiacal honey," this East Indian native and sacred fruit is a symbol for love. Mango leaves are hung as wedding decorations to enhance fertility, and the fruit is eaten by Indian men to improve their performance in bed. According to legend, Buddha found tranquility and rest in a mango grove. This fruit is sweet, juicy, and nearly impossible to eat without dribbling. Plus, it's very high in nutrients that boost sexual vitality, including vitamins C and A.

Oranges. Considered an expensive treat during the Sung Dynasty in China, where they were symbolically cut open and shared by lovers before sex, oranges have long been regarded as a symbol for love. To ensure a passionate union, ancient lovers bathed together in orange-scented water after having sex for the first time. Oranges were given as gifts to newlyweds to increase fertility, and courtesans perfumed their bedrooms with orange blossoms, a symbol of virginity and purity. An eighteenth-century love potion called Angel Water was made by combining orange blossom water with myrtle, rosewater, musk, and ambergris.

Lichee Nuts. A popular Chinese aphrodisiac that was once delivered to the emperor's concubines to keep them happy, this small brown fruit with red spikes, white interior, and a prune- or plume-like taste is now becoming more available in the United States. (Look for fresh, dried, and canned lichees in Chinese markets.) A similar fruit called logans, which have a rich, smoky flavor, is used in traditional Chinese medicine as a sex tonic.

When it comes to fruit, remember our favorite culinary acronym, K.I.S.S.: Keep it simple, sweetheart! Perfectly ripe fruit requires no preparation other than perhaps peeling, slicing, and maybe removing a few seeds. A selection of juicy fruits makes a perfect light dessert, snack, or brunch. To make your aphrodisiac experience more exciting, experiment with exotic fruits you have never

cheese please: fruit's perfect foil

Lovers and gourmets have always enjoyed cheese served as an appetizer or after dinner with dried or perfectly ripe fruit. Cheese is smooth, silky, sensuous, and delicious, perfect for romantic refueling and the perfect foil for juicy fruits. Plus it's energizing, protein rich, and a great source of calcium.

Always serve cheeses at room temperature. For a perfect cheese course, pick three or four different cheeses with contrasting textures, flavors, and colors such as American cheddar, a perfectly ripe Brie or Camembert, and a smoked Gouda. The choice depends on your own personal preference. Going out to eat? Invite your date home for a cheese course and a little post-prandial amour.

tasted or try exotic varieties of familiar fruits. Follow these rules whenever possible:

1. A peach grown on a local farm or neighbor's tree in August tastes much better than one shipped halfway around the world in December, so try to buy fruit in season and as close to its source as possible.
2. Heavy fruits are generally juicy fruits, so look for fruit that appears heavy for its size.
3. Seize the moment and eat your fruit at the peak of ripeness. (You can speed up the ripening process by placing fruit in a sealed paper bag. To really speed up the process, add a banana.) Get to know individual fruits to determine when they are best.

If your fruit lacks flavor even after you follow our advice, fear not. There are a number of aphrodisiacs to add and methods to use at your disposal to enliven a blackened banana, bruised peach, or limp fig. Here are our top ten ways to deal with less-than-perfect fruit.

10. Freeze with ease. Purée fruit (enough to make about 2 cups purée) with about ¼ cup sugar that has been dissolved in 1 cup warm juice or wine and some aphrodisiacs (try mint, basil, or a dash of cayenne). Freeze mixture in ice cube trays. When you are ready to serve, purée mixture in a blender for a wonderful sorbet.

9. Don't toss it unless it's into a salad. Cut up fruit, soak in a little lemon or lime juice to prevent browning, and mix with aphrodisiacal nuts and herbs; serve as a salad. Fruit wedges dipped in finely chopped herbs make a nice garnish.

8. Add a little zest. Slice fruit and toss with citrus juice and orange zest.

7. It's a snap. Top sliced fruit with a little whipped cream and either crystallized ginger (chopped) or crumbled ginger snaps. Or make a fruit crisp or cobbler by placing cut up fruit in a baking dish; covering with sweetened biscuit dough or a mixture of ½ cup oatmeal, ½ cup flour, ½ cup brown sugar, ¼ cup butter, and ¼ cup nuts; and baking at 350° F for about 30 minutes.

6. Make a compote by simmering or baking peeled and pared fruit with sugar, honey, or maple syrup and spices such as cinnamon, allspice, and nutmeg. Eat plain or use as a spicy crepe filling.

5. Steep or poach cut-up fruit in wine and spices.

4. Make flambé. Heat 2 to 3 tablespoons butter with 2 to 3 tablespoons brown sugar over low heat for about 5 minutes. Add sliced fruit and sauté until tender. Add 2 ounces of liqueur and ignite.

3. Toss fruit with whipped cream and sweeten with sugar to taste.

2. Purée fruit (this works well with berries) with a little cream and sugar to taste. Use as a dessert sauce or mix it with vanilla ice cream and refreeze.

1. Dip it good, in chocolate, that is. Make a fondue by melting chocolate chips in the microwave or in a double boiler. Or

make a spicy fruit dip by melting ⅓ cup hot pepper jelly in the microwave and mixing with 3 tablespoons honey and 1 cup yogurt or sour cream.

Fruit is nature's candy and sweet libido fuel, any way you slice it!

The Cooking Couple's Juicy Fruit Menu for Amour

{ Aphro Fruit Salsa }

Serve with tortilla chips, grilled fish, or chicken.

1 small ripe papaya; peeled, seeded, and diced into ¼-inch squares

1 small ripe mango; peeled, seeded, and diced into ¼-inch squares

1 medium ripe avocado; peeled, seeded, and diced into ¼-inch squares

¼ cup minced red onion

¼ cup fresh cilantro, chopped

¼ cup lime juice

2 jalapeño peppers, minced

1 teaspoon grated fresh gingerroot

Salt to taste

Combine all ingredients in a medium nonreactive bowl. Cover and refrigerate until ready to serve. Serve cool or at room temperature.

{ Summer Fruit Soup }

Served as either a first course or a light, refreshing dessert, this is a delicious way to enjoy summer's sexy bounty.

4 cups grape juice (white, red, or a mixture of both)

⅓ cup sugar

Juice of one lemon

1 teaspoon vanilla extract

4 cups mixed summer fruit (peaches, nectarines, and plums), pitted and coarsely chopped into 1- to 2-inch pieces

1 cup berries (blackberries, raspberries, or sliced strawberries)

Mint leaves for garnish

In a large bowl or soup tureen combine grape juice, sugar, lemon juice, and vanilla extract. Stir well to dissolve sugar. Add chopped fruit and berries and chill until serving time. Serve soup garnished with mint leaves and kisses.

Serves 4

{ Fruit Tart }

Quick, easy, and guaranteed to impress your sweet-tart. This recipe works well with apples, pears, and peaches. You can also try it with 1½ cups berries.

2 to 3 pieces medium ripe fruit

1 tablespoon lemon juice

2 tablespoons sugar

1 sheet frozen puff pastry (from a 17¼-ounce package), thawed

1 tablespoon fruit jelly

1. Preheat oven to 375° F.

2. Peel, core, and slice fruit ⅛-inch thick. In a small nonreactive bowl, toss sliced fruit with the lemon juice and sugar and set aside.

3. Using a floured rolling pin and work surface, roll out puff pastry sheet into an 11 x 7-inch rectangle.

4, Place on lightly greased baking sheet. Form a border around tart by folding up all 4 edges of the pastry about ¾ of an inch.

5. Fill pastry with overlapping fruit slices.

6. Bake until pastry edges are golden-brown, about 25 minutes.

7. Melt jelly or jam in microwave and brush over cooked tart.

Serves 6

{ Baked Love Apples }

A simple dessert or nice brunch dish that can be served hot or cold. Try experimenting with different aphrodisiac fillings. Ginger (crystallized or powdered), cloves, nutmeg, allspice, raisins, and dried figs all work well.

4 large, tart apples

¼ cup brown sugar

2 tablespoons butter

2 tablespoons chopped nuts

1 teaspoon ground cinnamon

⅛ teaspoon cardamom

1. Preheat oven to 350° F.
2. Using an apple corer remove core of apples, leaving about ½ an inch at the bottom of each apple. Place apples in a small roasting pan.
3. Combine sugar, butter, nuts, cinnamon, and cardamom. Place about 2 tablespoons of the mixture inside each apple and pour ½ cup water into roasting pan.
4. Bake, basting occasionally with pan juices, until apples are tender, about 20 minutes.

Serves 4

{ Fruit Pilaf }

A unique side dish that works well with meat or poultry or as part of a vegetarian meal. Look for bulgur wheat in health food stores or stores that carry Middle Eastern foods. You can also substitute 3 cups cooked rice for the bulgur and water or broth.

1½ cups uncooked bulgur wheat

2 cups hot water or broth (vegetable or chicken)

1 tablespoon olive oil

1 medium onion, chopped

2 cups dried mixed fruit (apples, figs, apricots, peaches, and prunes all work well), chopped

½ teaspoon ground cinnamon

Dash nutmeg

½ teaspoon ground cloves

Salt and freshly ground black pepper to taste

1. Combine bulgur wheat and hot water or broth in a bowl. Cover and set aside until liquid is absorbed, about 20 minutes.
2. Sauté onion in oil until soft, about 5 minutes.
3. Toss cooked bulgur wheat with remaining ingredients and serve.

Serves 4 as a side dish

Fruit Aphro-snacks

{ Basic smoothie }

A great quick energy drink. Feel free to experiment with your favorite juicy fruits.

1 ripe banana

1 cup berries, 1 ripe mango, or 1 peach (peeled and seeded)

1 cup milk or fruit juice

1 cup ice cubes

Place all ingredients in a blender and blend until smooth.

Serves 2

{ Avocado coffee Frappe }

We know this sounds like a strange combination, but this Indonesian beverage is creamy and delicious. Try serving it over ice or, for a frosty thicker version, blend the ice right in. Make enough for two or you will fight over who gets to drink it.

½ medium ripe avocado, peeled and pitted

1½ cups cold black coffee

⅓ cup sweetened condensed milk

1½ cups ice cubes

Optional flavor shots: 2 teaspoons vanilla extract, 2 tablespoons chocolate sauce, or 2 shots coffee liqueur.

Combine avocado, coffee, milk, and optional flavor shots in a blender and blend until smooth. Either serve over ice or add ice to blender and blend until smooth, about 1 minute.

Serves 2

{ Fruit cocktail }

4 ounces pear nectar

3 ounces Metaxa (Greek brandy)

1 ounce crème de rose

1 tablespoon honey

2 tablespoons fig jam

Blend all ingredients in a cocktail shaker filled with ice. To serve, strain into two martini glasses rimmed with honey.

Serves 2

{ Banana s'mores }

2 bananas

2 tablespoons chocolate chips

1 tablespoon miniature marshmallows

4 graham cracker squares

Remove a 1-inch-wide strip of peel from each banana. Using a small, sharp knife cut a ½-inch-wide by ¼-inch-deep strip of fruit the length of the banana. Fill each banana with half the chocolate chips and half the marshmallows. Wrap each individual banana in foil and bake in toaster oven at 350° F until chocolate and marshmallows melt, about 15 minutes. Unwrap bananas and let cool so they can be easily handled. Remove peels. Cut bananas into ½-inch slices and sandwich slices between graham crackers.

Serves 2

7

Lovable Lilies and Amorous Alliums

Pictures of Lily, made my life so wonderful. . . .

—Pete Townshend, The Who

You have to kiss a lot of frogs to find a handsome prince—or beautiful princess. Fortunately, there are plenty of lovable lilies, many of which are aphrodisiacs, to pad your way as you hop from breakfast to lunch to dinner. You may not find your true love with the first kiss, but with the help of these three edible lilies—garlic, onion, and asparagus—you'll have a great time searching.

Allium Encounters of the Third Kind

Shallots are for lovers; onions are for men; garlic is for heroes.

—unknown

The lily family, *Liliaceae* to you Latin lovers, is one of the largest plant families, with about 3,500 species worldwide. Most are ornamental flowering plants, such as tulips and hyacinths, but some, like onions, garlic, leeks, shallots, and asparagus, are vegetables and renowned aphrodisiacs, constantly appearing in both European and Asian erotic literature.

Allium Allures

General Ulysses S. Grant demanded, "I will not move my army without onions!" Hall of Fame baseball great Ted Williams said, "I

Monet's Muse

Water lilies are not lilies. Made famous by the French impressionist painter Claude Monet, water lilies are members of the Nymphaeaceae family. *Nymphae* means "inner lips of the vulva" and is the root of the word *nymphomaniac,* meaning "a woman with excessive sexual desires."

Of course, this is subjective. After all, one person's "excessive" is another person's "great date."

can't get enough garlic." And everybody's favorite fiddler, Emperor Nero, consumed so many leeks to improve his performance in bed *and* his singing voice (think Elvis in a toga) that people called him *porrophages* ("leek-eater") behind his back. According to legend, those who uttered this phrase too near the emperor's ear generally lost theirs.

In the scandalous seduction manual *The Art of Love,* the Roman writer Ovid recommended shallots as an aphrodisiac. In the Bible's Book of Numbers the Israelites complained to Moses about the foods they left behind: "We remember the fish, which we did eat in Egypt freely; the cucumbers, the melons, the leeks, the onions, and the garlic." All aphrodisiacs!

Cooking without alliums is like having sex without kissing. It can be done, but the result lacks sweetness, depth, and passion. Alliums are standard residents in our kitchen. Onions, garlic, and the other members of the allium (*allium* is Latin for "garlic") family—leeks, shallots, scallions, and chives—provide the simple, sweet savoriness that anchors erotic cuisine while elevating it to the height of edible ecstasy.

Treat alliums right and they will make your taste buds sing even while bringing tears to your eyes.

The Stinking Rose

There is no such thing as a little garlic.

–Arthur Baer, American journalist

The most renowned and powerful member of the allium family is garlic, aka the stinking rose. Like Danny DeVito, he's the small assertive type who takes a bit of getting used to before you fall in love.

You probably won't want to kiss him on the first date, but once you get a taste, you will fall head over cloves for this hunk of flavor. We agree with author Leo Buscaglia, who said: "There are many miracles in the world to be celebrated, and for me, garlic is among the most deserving." Garlic is worthy of love, respect, and praise.

In the first half of the twentieth century, garlic had not yet become popular on the American culinary scene, and was ignorantly ridiculed by bigots as "Italian perfume." Dr. William J. Robinson, an eminent New York gynecologist, popular writer on health, and early advocate of birth control, wrote: "There is one spice or condiment about which I hesitate to speak because it is held in such contempt and disdain in this country. I refer to garlic. There can be no question as to its pronounced aphrodisiac effect. In fact, it stands at the head of the list. But many Anglo-Saxons would perhaps prefer their impotence to the alternative of having to eat garlic."

The Egyptians, Chinese, Japanese, Jews, Greeks, Romans, and Europeans did not share the Anglo-Saxon bigotry against garlic. Asian lovers ate garlic to enhance sexual strength and beauty. The Romans consecrated garlic to Ceres (the goddess of agriculture), believed that eating garlic stimulated the penis, and made a love potion from pressed garlic juice.

Sacred to Hecate, the dark goddess of witches, garlic was also used in love potions and to reverse spells for impotence. In Elizabethan England, despite the prejudice against it, garlic was proclaimed an aphrodisiac believed to "reawaken spent desire." To enhance his sexiness and sexual performance, King Henry IV of France, who was baptized with a clove of garlic on his lips, ate copious quantities of garlic before sleeping with women.

From the days of Moses, Jews, who were called "garlic eaters," have had a love affair with the potent bulb. (You know why New York's Chinatown looks like downtown Tel Aviv on Saturday night? Because Jewish people have always loved Chinese food. Why? It contains copious amounts of garlic.)

In the fourth century B.C., the religious leader and reformer Ezra issued an order requiring Jews to eat garlic on Sabbath

Ancient Garlic Love Potions

In *Natural History*, the Roman naturalist Pliny the Elder listed over 60 different medical uses for garlic, from repelling serpents and scorpions to restoring passion. Although we live near the ocean, we're not too worried about repelling serpents. So here's some advice on arousal from Pliny and some other garlic lovers.

According to Pliny: "Pound a little garlic with fresh coriander and take it with some neat wine, and those sex problems will be gone."

From the *Kama Sutra*: "Mix garlic root with white pepper and licorice. When drunk with sugared milk, it enhances virility."

From *The Perfumed Garden*: "Men whose impotence is due either to the corruption of their sperm owing to their cold nature, or to maladies of the organs, or to discharges or fevers and similar ills, or to their excessive promptness in ejaculation, can be cured. They should eat stimulant pastry containing honey, ginger, pyrether, syrup of vinegar, hellebore, garlic, cinnamon, nutmeg, cardamoms, sparrows' tongues, Chinese cinnamon, long pepper, and other spices. They will be cured by using them."

nights because "it promotes love and arouses desire." According to the Talmud (the authoritative body of Jewish tradition), garlic was believed to increase passion and fertility and thus enhance marital lovemaking and procreation, important parts of observing the Sabbath. To this day garlic still plays a vital role in Jewish cooking, making an appearance in foods ranging from roast chicken to pickles.

Not every religion saw garlic as beneficial. In certain Eastern religions, garlic was banned by celibate monks, and the teachings of Buddhism forbid priests and other enlightenment seekers from eating garlic—as well as scallions, onions, shallots, and leeks—because of their stimulating power.

The pungent garlic bulb is legendary for its magical and medicinal powers, and has been used for everything from vanquishing vampires and demons to preventing the plague.

Ancient Egyptians worshiped garlic and used it as part of the embalming process. Believing in sex in the afterlife, they placed whole cloves in their tombs. (Gives a whole new meaning to "raising the dead.") They fed it to their slaves to keep them healthy and energized. (You need all the help you can get when you're dragging around two-ton rocks.) Before the days of steroids and other performance-enhancing concoctions, ancient Olympians ate garlic to increase strength and stamina.

Facts Behind the FolkLore

> *I cannot imagine life without garlic, and consider it one of the best general tonics for the healing system.*
>
> −Dr. Andrew weiL

Science is peeling away the myths surrounding garlic and revealing that under the papery skin lie chemicals that can enhance erections, lower cholesterol, and help prevent tumors.

Garlic is a scientifically proven aphrodisiac. Especially when

nature's viagra

The chemical and physiological reactions that garlic creates naturally in a man's body work along the same lines as Viagra.

During sexual arousal, a highly reactive gas called nitric oxide is released into the corpus cavernosum of the penis. Nitric oxide activates an enzyme called guanylate cyclase, which increases levels of cyclic guanosine monophosphate (cGMP), which relaxes and dilates blood vessels in the penis so that blood can flow, resulting in an erection.

The active ingredient in Viagra, sildenafil, boosts the effect of nitric oxide by blocking an enzyme that reduces nitric oxide levels. Garlic achieves a similar result by increasing the activity of nitric oxide synthase, the enzyme that makes nitric oxide from L-arginine.

In short, both Viagra and garlic work by increasing blood flow to the penis so an erection can be obtained by increasing levels of nitric oxide.

Let's face it. Garlic is cheaper, safer, and tastes better than some little blue pill that has possible side effects including headache, dizziness, blue-tinged vision, and diarrhea.

taken with the amino acid L-arginine, garlic can naturally increase blood levels of nitric oxide, a molecule that is essential for getting and maintaining an erection. (For more on L-arginine see Chapter 10, "The Cooking Couple's Best Sex Diet.") Garlic works by increasing the activity of an enzyme called nitric oxide synthase (NOS) so that more nitric oxide can be made from L-arginine.

A clove or two of garlic is particularly effective for people with low NOS levels, such as men over forty. (Middle-aged men usually show a drop in nitric oxide levels, which can lead to erectile dysfunction.) And even if your erections are rock hard, you may want to cash in on the side effects of raising nitric oxide levels with garlic, which include lowering blood pressure and preventing angina.

According to Varro E. Tyler, Ph.D., one of the leading authorities on herbal medicine, garlic and other alliums take the prize for the most popular herbal remedies of all time. The Garlic Information Center gives a long list of ills that can be treated with garlic, from athlete's foot to wasp stings.

Many studies show that garlic is a major hero to the circulatory system, and anything that significantly boosts blood circulation improves sexual vitality.

For people with high cholesterol (over 200), half to a whole clove of garlic per day helps keep the cardiologist away. According to a report published in the *Annals of Internal Medicine* summarizing the results of five studies on garlic's effect on blood cholesterol, garlic lowered total cholesterol levels by about 9 percent. A German study found garlic supplements decreased total cholesterol levels by 12 percent in only four weeks.

Like wine and aspirin, garlic also thins the blood, preventing clots. Plus, garlic stops bad LDL cholesterol from oxidizing and clogging veins and arteries, and studies suggest it can help lower blood pressure and blood sugar.

strong smell, strong medicine

Garlic's strong scent arises from a powerful chemical reaction. When a garlic clove is cut, its cells release an enzyme called allinaise that transforms an odorless chemical called alliin into a

Flashing

By the way, it's not just humans who use nitric oxide (NO) in the sexual arena. Fireflies, who flash to find a mate, use nitric oxide to trigger the light-producing reaction.

Dispelling the Smell

When you eat garlic (or rub it on your skin) allicin is absorbed into the blood and lungs; as a result, your body and breath smell like garlic. While the only way to rid yourself completely of the smell is to stop eating garlic, munching on a little parsley (another sexual stimulant), chewing on a citrus peel, or rinsing your mouth with water mixed with lemon juice can help.

But hey, what's a little garlic odor in return for lower cholesterol, better circulation, and harder erections? "I'll take the scampi, please."

strong-smelling sulfur-containing molecule called allicin, which is what makes garlic so valuable medicinally.

The mineral sulfur, which is found in garlic as well as onions, asparagus, and eggs, is required for the production of glutathione, an antioxidant found in all living cells that helps protect the body from toxins and premature aging.

According to researchers at Penn State, to increase the formation of disease-preventing substances in garlic, let your minced or crushed garlic sit for at least 10 minutes before eating so the allicin has plenty of time to form.

One of the few herbs used in all three major healing systems (Western, traditional Chinese, and Ayurvedic), the mighty bulb is a powerful antibiotic that was used in both world wars as an antiseptic. Garlic also kills viruses that cause colds and flu. Taken internally, garlic boosts the immune system by stimulating T-cells, and human and animal studies show it helps prevent cancers on three levels.

·It detoxifies carcinogens (substances that produce or incite cancer).

·It prevents normal, healthy cells from becoming cancerous.

·It directly inhibits cancerous cells from growing.

According to researchers at the Byrd Health Science Center at West Virginia University, garlic's "broad range of beneficial effects are worthy of serious consideration in clinical trials for the prevention and treatment of cancer."

Pregnant women may want to add a clove or two of garlic to their daily diet. Preliminary studies show that garlic may help prevent complications of pregnancy including preeclampsia

The Vampire's Kiss

The Sanskrit word for garlic translates as "slayer of monsters." In Eastern Europe and the Mediterranean, particularly Italy, garlic was considered excellent protection against evil. According to the Roman poet Virgil, garlic kept Circe from changing Ulysses into a pig like his companions. Garlic's age-old reputation as protection against evil has translated into the modern belief that it wards off vampires.

Today, some practitioners of ancient Wicca (or witchcraft) eat garlic to guard themselves from evil and ill health. Some mountain climbers carry garlic to ward off bad weather, and people traveling over water may take a clove with them to prevent drowning. The Sherpas of Nepal (home of Mount Everest) recommend garlic soup as a remedy for altitude sickness. Here are some other creatures of the day and night that garlic purportedly wards off.

Vampire bats. In Panama, people rub garlic on their feet to keep the bats from biting.

Horses. Jockeys in Hungary place garlic on their horses' bits to keep the competition from passing them.

Bugs. Garlic is used throughout the world to protect crops from insects, and as a mosquito repellent.

Rabbits and deer. Scientists at the University of Washington found garlic placed around trees keeps animals away.

Bulls. Matadors wear garlic around their necks for protection.

Roses for Romance

Full of love she [the rose] is Aphrodite's servant; with fragrant leaves shining brilliantly she sways above the foliage, bathing in the smiles of Zephyr.

—Achilles Tatius, Greek rhetorician and author

While garlic is a member of the lily family, its pet name is the stinking rose. Sacred to the goddess of love, Venus, roses are the most amorous flower. According to legend, Venus's son Cupid bribed Harpocrates, the god of silence, with a rose to keep his mother's love affairs quiet.

- To seduce Mark Antony, Cleopatra carpeted an entire room with rose petals so that the scent would engulf him.
- Roses fueled so many Roman orgies that the flower became a symbol of the decadence of the emperors. At one party thrown by Emperor Elagabalus, a number of guests actually suffocated under tons of roses.
- Nero decorated a banquet hall with thousands of roses and released a flock of rose-scented pigeons above his guests. The Romans filled their fountains with rose water and used rose oil in cosmetics.
- Persian women used roses as a love charm to win back straying lovers.
- In colonial America, women kept their men interested by serving them rose-flavored brandy.
- To stimulate romance, Chinese lovers still drink a mixture of prunes, sugar, olives, and rose petals.

Roses, tasty and nutritious, have been eaten for thousands of years. Here are some easy ways to incorporate roses into your diet and life.

- Sprinkle fruit or green salads with a few petals (make sure they have been grown without pesticides).

- Eat candied roses. You can make these by dipping rose petals in egg white, then sugar, and letting them dry on wax paper.
- Add a few drops of rose water to beverages, frozen desserts, or whipped cream. Look for rose water in stores that sell Middle Eastern foods.
- Toss a few rose petals between the sheets and let their aroma work its wonders.
- Give each other a rose facial.

{ Rose FaciaL }

¼ cup torn rose petals
½ cup ground oatmeal (You can grind it in the blender.)
¼ cup honey

Mix the torn rose petals with the oatmeal and then the honey. Wash your faces, pat the mixture on your lover's face, and relax in a rose-scented bath (use either additional rose petals, rose water, or rose essential oil) together for 30 minutes. Rinse each other off with warm water and a washcloth. To keep the glow going and get your endorphins jumping, try an erotic massage with rose-scented oil (combine 2 to 3 drops rose essential oil with 3 ounces of almond oil). Check out page 118 for details.

(high blood pressure during pregnancy), preterm labor, and growth retardation. Plus, babies really groove on garlic. According to a study published in the journal *Pediatrics,* when nursing women eat garlic, their babies drink more breast milk. Nutritionally, garlic also contains calcium as well as vitamin C and is low in calories.

A Pungent History

Garlic, the herb of Mars (the Roman god of war), has been lending its supernatural, medicinal, and aphrodisiacal powers to humans for eons and is one of mankind's oldest and probably one of its first cultivated plant foods.

There are several myths about garlic's origin. According to an Indian legend, garlic sprang from the blood of Ruhu after the god Vishnu beheaded him for stealing and drinking the elixir of life. The prophet Muhammad claimed that garlic sprouted from the ground where Satan placed his left foot as he left the Garden of Eden, and onions sprouted from the ground under his right. Muhammad said nothing about the origin of chicken wings.

More than three hundred different varieties of garlic are cultivated today, all of which probably originated in Central Asia or the Eastern Mediterranean. The wide variety of names for garlic, its pervasive use in ancient cultures, and its even wider use in modern society illustrate the importance that society places on the bulb as a food, medicine, and aphrodisiac.

The English word *garlic* came either from the Welsh *garlleg* or from the Anglo-Saxon *gar-leac, gar* meaning "spear" and *leac* meaning "leek."

Releasing the Magic

Garlic is an essential ingredient in many cuisines, particularly Asian and Mediterranean. We never run out of fresh garlic, and neither should you. Here are the basics you need to know to buy, store, and prepare garlic.

Buying. Garlic is a seasonal crop, and 80 to 90 percent of the garlic Americans eat comes from California. The flavor is best during the first few months after harvest in the summer and early fall. Select heads that are firm to the touch and free from dark spots, which indicate mold.

Storage. If properly stored, garlic will keep for two to three months. The heads are happiest when housed unpeeled, in a cool, dark place, in an open container or in a garlic pot with holes. Don't refrigerate; cold decreases garlic's flavor. When little green sprouts (which have a bitter taste) appear, it means your garlic is starting to deteriorate and should be used quickly.

Usage. While you can buy peeled or minced garlic, freshly prepared garlic has the best flavor and is chemically most effective.

Peeling cloves is easy. Simply separate a clove from the rest of the head. Place it on a cutting board and smash it with the flat side of a chef's knife or cleaver by pressing down quickly and firmly on the knife with your hand (this also enlivens garlic's flavor). The clove will crack, the skin will easily slip off, and voilá, you're ready to chop garlic like a pro.

To chop or mince garlic, use a chef's knife to make several slices (the long way) in your peeled clove. Then cut across the clove. To finish the job, make rocking motions with your knife across the cut garlic until you obtain the desired mince. You can also use a press or grater. Because the press breaks more garlic cells, resulting in a stronger flavor, use this method when you want a very powerful garlic presence.

Another option, which produces fabulous flavor, is to crush a clove or two of garlic with a little coarse salt and mix into a paste using a mortar and pestle. Add other aphrodisiacal herbs and spices such as basil, ginger, or parsley for an erotically arousing rub that can be spread on meat, chicken, or fish prior to cooking.

For less-pronounced, mellower garlic flavor, add whole cloves to stews and soups or rub whole cloves inside baking dishes, sauté pans, or salad bowls. Whole cloves can also be roasted of grilled and served alongside meats or vegetables.

garlic divides, garlic conquers

Garlicks, tho' used by the French, are better adapted to the uses of medicine than cookery.

—amelia simmons, author, *american cookery,*
the first cookbook to be published
in the united states, 1796

Garlic was not always an ingredient on the American cuisine scene. Derided as "Bronx vanilla" because so many Italians settled there after immigrating in the late nineteenth and early twentieth centuries, until recently garlic was considered a crude food fit only for immigrants and the working class. Then along came eminent American food writer James Beard, hailed as the "father of American cooking," who introduced America to the joys of garlic in the 1950s when he presented a Provençal recipe called Chicken with 40 Cloves of Garlic on television's first cooking show.

Americans have learned a trick or two from the French since Amelia Simmons maligned garlic in 1796—one is how to French kiss, and the other is to love garlic. Today, U.S. garlic consump-

"Hey, garlic breath, you're busted!"

In some towns, under certain circumstances, garlic breath is illegal. In Alexandria, Minnesota, a man cannot make love to his wife with the smell of garlic, onions, or sardines on his breath. In Gary, Indiana, it is against the law to go to the theater within four hours of eating garlic.

Have you ever noticed how odd things keep coming out of Gary, Indiana? Well, it is Michael Jackson's hometown, after all.

Five Easy Ways to Make
Garlic Part of Your Love Life

1. Use roasted garlic like butter, as a bread spread or flavoring for soups, dips, and mashed potatoes. To roast a head of garlic, trim the tops off the cloves, drizzle with olive oil, season with salt and pepper, wrap in foil, and bake at 350° F until soft, about 45 minutes. Let cool, then squeeze the now-creamy cloves out of their skin.

2. Tuck sliced garlic cloves under chicken skin before you bake, roast, or grill it. Or make slits in meat or fish and place slivered garlic in holes. (This is a great way to flavor leg of lamb.)

3. Rub bread with a cut clove of garlic to flavor it before toasting or using for sandwiches. Or cut a baguette into 1/4-inch-thick slices and rub the slices with the cut side of a garlic clove. Place slices on a rimmed baking dish, sprinkle with Parmesan cheese, and bake at 350° F, until golden brown, about 10 minutes. Serve like crackers with cheese or soup.

4. Make a batch of pesto and toss with pasta, spread on bread, or use as a topping for sautéed chicken breasts or grilled tuna steaks.

5. Add raw or sautéed minced garlic to soups, stews, and spaghetti sauce.

{ Pesto }

2 cups fresh basil leaves, washed and dried
6 cloves fresh garlic
1/2 cup pine nuts
2/3 cup coarsely grated Parmesan
2/3 cup extra virgin olive oil
Salt and pepper to taste
Combine basil, garlic, pine nuts, and Parmesan in a blender or food processor. With the motor running, slowly add the olive oil. Store in the refrigerator or place in ice cube trays and freeze for later use.

tion continues to rise. In 1919 per capita consumption was under one ounce. From 1989 to 1999, annual consumption increased from 1 to 3.1 pounds per person.

Thanks to garlic champions like Italian immigrants and food writers like James Beard and, of course, Julia Child, garlic has conquered America. Today, there are designer garlics with fancy names like Silverskin, Persian Star, and Mootka Rose, specifically bred for their unique flavor, strength, and/or appearance. The wonder food is gaining ever more attention and respect in culinary, medical, and aphrodisiacal circles. In the words of James Beard, garlic is "something that no good cook can live without." And, we might add, no good lover *should* be without.

onions: Beauty is more than skin Deep

If your wife is old and your member is exhausted, eat onions in plenty.

—Martial, the Roman epigrammatist

From the Cheops Pyramid to the battlefields of the Civil War, the onion has been eaten to increase valor, strength, and sperm production. Like garlic, the humble onion, one of the world's oldest cultivated foods, was used by many ancient peoples as an aphrodisiac and medicinal herb.

While the rest of their society ate and worshiped onions (which were a symbol for eternity and used, like the Bible, for taking oaths), Egyptian priests abstained to help them stay chaste. Asian aphrodisiacal dishes frequently contain onions. The Greeks and Romans ate onions, which are ruled by the masculine planet Mars, to improve sexual endurance as well as valor in battle. And, as part of ancient Greek marriage rituals, the bride would give her new husband a basket of onions at the conclusion of the marriage ceremony.

What chicken soup is to the common cold, onion soup is to a

weary libido. Like garlic, onions improve sexual vitality by en-hancing blood circulation, and according to Indian herbalist H. K. Bakhru, as an aphrodisiac, onions are second only to garlic in their ability to increase the libido and strengthen the repro-ductive organs in both sexes.

If you're too tired for sex, onions can help revitalize you. Too timid to make the first move? Bite into an onion for the courage and strength to pounce. Want to give an Olympic performance in bed? Train like the ancient Greeks, who prepared for athletic com-petitions by eating pounds of onions chased by onion juice and an onion body massage. Or take the advice of the first-century

Q is for quercetin

Onions are a nutritious, low-calorie way to flavor dishes. They con-tain healthy doses of vitamin C, folic acid, potassium, and fiber, and are a great source of disease-preventing phytochemicals.

Scientists are particularly intrigued by a phytochemical in onions called quercetin. Also found in tea and apples, quercetin is an an-tioxidant that prevents damage in cells and tissues. Studies show that quercetin inhibits the oxidization of LDL cholesterol, which can lead to atherosclerosis and heart disease, and it eliminates free rad-icals, and boosts the protective effects of vitamin E. Research is showing that quercetin may also help prevent cataracts, as well as a number of cancers.

Here are some other healthy facts about onions.

•Eating onions may prevent gastric ulcers.

•According to studies done at the University of Wisconsin, Madison, pungent onions exhibit strong anti-platelet activity, and may therefore reduce the risk of stroke and heart disease.

•A Swiss study conducted at the University of Bern suggests that onions may help prevent osteoporosis.

Roman horticulturist Columella, who declared, "Onions inflame and enliven girls." Any way you slice, dice, or chop them, onions and your libido should be buddies.

The French were on to something when they invented onion soup. It's so popular that it is served in the lowest bistro as well as the most celebrated four-star restaurant, and so potent that it is traditionally enjoyed by newlyweds the morning after their wedding to reinvigorate romance.

In South Africa couples keep their honeymoon humming by eating an onion and singing a song before bed. (T. Rex's "Get It On (Bang a Gong)" seems to be most popular.)

Guatemalan men eat onions to remain virile and fertile as they age.

onion Love Potions

From east, west, north, and south, ancient cultures all seemed to believe that onions opened the door to amatory bliss.

Sheikh Nefzaoui, author of *The Perfumed Garden*, gives several aphrodisiacal recipes using onions. He recommends eating pounded onion seed mixed with honey while fasting. Nefzaoui also suggests drinking a mixture made of one part onion juice and two parts honey that has been heated to evaporate some of the liquid. (The sheikh cautions the reader to use the honey-onion mixture sparingly, no more than three days in a row.) Nefzaoui also says eating fried onions and egg yolks with condiments for a few days will result in "surpassing and invaluable vigor for the coitus."

Here's an earlier Arabic recipe to create sexual desire: Boil onions with green beans and spice with cardamom, cinnamon, and ginger.

"For those who seek the door of love," the Roman Marcus Terentius Varro (aka Reatimus) recommends stimulating the libido by eating a mixture of cooked onions combined with pine nuts (another renowned aphrodisiac), mustard, and pepper.

The Greek physician Galen, like Sheikh Nefzaoui, also suggests consuming honey mixed with onions. Another fan of the pine nut, Galen recommends a bedtime snack of pine nuts, honey, and almonds.

Ovid, author of *Remedia Amoris,* suggests "onions and snails' heads without sauce." C'mon, Ovid, who would be stupid enough to ruin a good snail's head with sauce?

According to Indian herbalist H. K. Bakhru, the white variety of onion should be peeled, crushed, and fried in pure butter. This mixture acts as an excellent aphrodisiac tonic if taken regularly with a spoon of honey on an empty stomach. The powder of black gram (a type of dal or legume used in Indian cooking), when dipped in onion juice then dried, produces a mixture called *kanji.* This also acts as an aphrodisiac.

The Aztecs made a sauce called *ahuaca-mulli,* the predecessor of our guacamole, from mashed avocado, tomatoes, and onions, all of which are aphrodisiacs.

Jamaica is famous for its wet jerk rub (this is not a reference to Jerry Lewis's hair), which is often made from onion juice, along with other aphrodisiacs including chile peppers, cinnamon, garlic, and nutmeg. Enjoy some jerked pork or chicken with an Irish moss rum cocktail (Irish moss is a well-known Jamaican aphrodisiac made from the gelatinous extract of seaweed) or a Guinness beer, and you'll be singing all the way to the beach.

The onion's elusive origins

While the exact origins of the onion are hard to trace, food historians, archeologists, and botanists generally believe the onion, which was a staple food for prehistoric man, sprang up in central Asia. Easy to grow and store, onions were first cultivated in the Middle East at least 5,000 years ago. The Jews were so fond of onions that they named a city constructed in 173 B.C., near the Gulf of Suez, Onion.

By the Middle Ages, onions, along with cabbage and beans, were one of the three main vegetables consumed in Europe. Eaten by both the rich and the poor, onions were given as wedding gifts, accepted as payment for rent, and used in folk medicine to treat headaches, gout, snakebites, coughs, congestion, and baldness. The Pilgrims took bulbs with them on the Mayflower, and when they arrived in America they found the Indians were already eating wild onions. In fact, one theory holds that Chicago was named for the local Indian word for wild onions, *chicago.*

Yellow onions are considered to have the most aphrodisiacal power and make up more than three quarters of the world's production. White onions are milder and moister than yellow onions. Reds (also called Bermuda) are the sweetest and mildest onion, and are the best of the bunch in recipes requiring onions in the raw.

Yellow, white, and red onions are available all year long. These days you can also find a variety of trendy sweet onions during the spring and summer such as Vidalia, Walla Walla, and Texas 1015. High in sugar and low in sulfur, some are so sweet that they can be eaten raw like apples.

After lettuce and potatoes, onions are the third most consumed fresh vegetable in America. Each year the United States grows over two million metric tons, and per capita consumption is over 18.3 pounds. The average world consumption is 13.67 pounds per person. Who loves onions the most? Libyans, who annually eat 66.8 pounds per person.

onion 101

Here's what you need to know to keep onions in your passion-filled pantry.

Buying. There are two types of onions, fresh and storage. Fresh onions (also called green onions, which are not the same as scallions) have a fresher, livelier flavor than storage onions and appear in the spring, summer, and early fall with their greens still attached. They are more delicate than storage onions and perish more readily. Look for fresh onions that are firm and free of cuts and blemishes.

Most of the onions we buy are storage onions—harvested in the fall and stored for year-round sale. Select regular onions that are blemish-free and hard (an indication of crispness) with short necks and dry, shiny, papery skins.

Storing. Fresh green onions should be stored in plastic bags in the refrigerator.

Regular yellow, white, and red storage onions should be kept in a single layer in a cool, dry place with good air circulation. If your onions sprout, it means the storage area is too warm. Mold means the area is too damp. Halved onions should be stored in the vegetable drawer of your refrigerator in a tightly closed plastic bag.

Slicing and dicing. The best way to cut onions is to split them in half from stem to root end and peel. Then place the flat half of the onion on a cutting board and cut horizontal slices from the stem to the root end. For a nice dice, make a series of crosscuts.

other ALLium encounters

Leeks

These alliums were used in Greek love potions, and the Romans considered them superior to onions and garlic. During the Middle Ages people ate leeks as an aphrodisiac, believing that they increased sperm count and enhanced the libido, especially when eaten with honey, almonds, and sesame seeds.

In the seventh century, leeks became the national symbol for Wales as Welsh warriors wore leeks in their hats in a decisive battlefield victory over the Saxons.

No More Tears

The tears that so frequently accompany onion preparation are caused by sulfuric compounds that are released in the air and irritate the eyes when onions are cut. A number of suggestions have been proposed to stop the tears, including:

- Use a sharp knife.
- Chill the onions for a few hours before cutting.
- Don't trim the root end, where the sulfur compounds are most intense, until the last possible moment.
- Rinse onions in water after you peel and cut them in half.
- Stand away from the cutting board when you slice and dice.
- Wear glasses.
- If all else fails, Michael recommends sticking your head in the freezer and breathing deeply through the nose. He swears it works.

Formally known as poor man's asparagus, today leeks are expensive due to the intensive labor and extensive time needed to grow them. Unlike garlic, onions, and shallots (which can be stored unrefrigerated for an extended period of time), leeks are always eaten soon after harvesting (either raw or cooked). Although they are available all year long, leek harvest peaks in the autumn.

The subtle, soft, sweet, yet full flavor of leeks is essential to the classic French cold soup vichyssoise, and is a wonderful addition to other soups, stews, and savory vegetable pies such as quiche. They can be braised, roasted, sautéed, or grilled and used to accent vegetable, rice, and meat dishes. With the exception of soups, most recipes call for using just the white part of the leek.

Buy leeks that are firm, with long, white necks, and avoid ones with large, swollen bulbs—an indication that the leek is too mature and may taste woody. Make sure to wash them well; dirt collects between the leaves as leeks grow.

Scallions

A key ingredient in Asian cuisines, these alliums are available throughout the year but are most abundant in the spring. Both the white and green parts can be eaten. Because scallions cook quickly, they are a great addition to stir-fries. They also can be sliced and used raw as a garnish or a flavoring for soups and egg dishes. Select scallions with bright and fresh (not wilted) greens, and trim the hairy white ends before use.

Shallots

These alliums are loved throughout the world, especially in the Mediterranean. In France, shallots are poached in wine and served alongside meat, and are used both raw and cooked in sauces such as mignonette (a dipping sauce for shellfish made from raw shallots and vinegar) and Bernaise, which is made from sautéed shallots and herbs. In Thailand and Cambodia thinly sliced shallots are fried quickly in oil and used as a garnish.

Buy shallots that are firm and store them as you would onions. If you can't find shallots, you can substitute a quarter of a small onion for each shallot.

Asparagus: The Most PhaLLic vegetable

A decoction of asparagus roots boiled in wine . . . stirreth up bodily lust in man and woman.

–NichoLas cuLpepper,
the seventeenth-century physician and
herbaList and author of *The EngLish Physician*

Tall, green, and handsome. Whether you like 'em thick or thin, that's what you get with this well-hung lily. One glance, and you know asparagus is definitely an aphrodisiac. The phallic stalks are an excellent example of the Doctrine of Signatures, an ancient medical theory that God (or the gods, depending on your religious orientation) created foods to resemble the purpose they were best suited for.

Because it looks like a penis, asparagus was and still is considered a psycho-physiological aphrodisiac, one that works by getting the mind to trigger a physiological response. Like oysters and figs (both of which resemble a vagina), walnuts (which resemble testicles), and other phallic foods such as cucumbers, carrots, and zucchini, asparagus work as an aphrodisiac because of their visual eroticism.

The most amorous asparagus lovers are the French. In fact, the French word for asparagus, *asperge*, is slang for "penis." During the Renaissance, asparagus was touted as an aphrodisiac and verboten in most convents. In the 1800s, French bridegrooms were required to eat several courses consisting of asparagus, asparagus, and more asparagus the night before their wedding because of its reputed powers to arouse. In the early part of the twentieth century several general-interest French magazines showed suggestive pictures of scantily clad women passionately hugging giant asparagus spears.

Asparagus contains compounds called steroid glycosides, which stimulate hormone production. The Chinese believe eating asparagus roots increases feelings of love and compassion. In the Middle East people make an aphrodisiac from boiled asparagus that has been fried and seasoned with condiments. The strange ammonia-like smell that many people notice in their urine after eating asparagus comes from two other chemicals, asparagusic acid and S-methylmethionine.

Asparagus is used as an herb in India to promote fertility, reduce menstrual cramping, and increase milk production in nursing mothers. To promote sexual vigor, the *Kama Sutra* also recommends drinking a paste made from asparagus and other ingredients. In the Middle East the vegetable is covered with egg yolk and eaten as an aphrodisiac. Some herbalists claim that as-

sarsapariLLa

Most people know sarsaparilla as a flavoring for root beer. Well, guess what? It also has a very lusty reputation as an aphrodisiac. A relative of wild asparagus, sarsaparilla (*Smilax officinalis*) is indigenous to the American Southeast, Mexico, and Central America. Mexican Indians used sarsaparilla root as a cure for impotence. Claims that sarsaparilla root contains testosterone are false, but it does contain steroids and saponins that may work like anabolic steroids, increasing the sex drive and the activity of the sex hormone testosterone. Sarsaparilla is often sold in formulas combined with other sexually stimulating herbs such as damiana, licorice, and muira-puama.

The herb was also used in Europe as far back as the sixteenth century as a cure for syphilis and other sexually transmitted diseases. Sarsaparilla is also a good general tonic herb that can increase overall wellness, stamina, and energy for both men and women.

paragus works as an aphrodisiac for men because it contains the chemical asparagine, a natural diuretic that stimulates the urinary tract and surrounding tissue.

Low in calories and high in vitamins A, C, and folic acid, asparagus, like onions and garlic, is rich in the immune-system-supporting antioxidant glutathione.

A Mediterranean native and one of the first crops ready for harvest in the spring, asparagus is a versatile vegetable. It can be eaten hot or cold, raw, steamed, boiled, sautéed, grilled, or roasted. It works well in salads, casseroles, and soups.

The bottom end of the asparagus stalk can be tough, so either snap off an inch or two from the stem end or peel away the tough outer skin with a vegetable peeler. (Peeling also results in more even cooking.) We like our asparagus with a little olive oil, lemon juice, fresh herbs, and salt and pepper. Don't dress your stalks

> ## staLking the staLks: thick or thin?
>
> The big debate is thick or thin. While big, thick stalks are meatier, thinner stalks are more tender and elegant on the plate. Both perform equally well, so the choice is really a matter of personal preference.

until the last minute. Acidic ingredients yellow the vegetable quickly.

Whatever way you decide to fix your stalks, remember, asparagus cooks quickly. It's done when it becomes tender and turns bright green.

Here's an asparagus tip from Madame de Pompadour, King Louis XV's mistress.

"Dress and cook the asparagus sticks in the normal way by plunging them into boiling water. Slice them obliquely toward the tips in pieces no bigger than the little finger. Take only the choicest sections, and keeping them hot, allow them to drain while the sauce is being prepared in the manner following—Work ten grammes of flour and a lump of butter together, a good pinch of powdered nutmeg and the yolks of two eggs diluted with four spoonfuls of water acidulated with lemon juice. After cooking this sauce, drop in the asparagus tips and serve in a covered casserole."

Allium encounters are erotic encounters, which is why the opening line of Laura Esquivel's *Like Water for Chocolate* illuminates the magical connection between alliums and romance: "Take care to chop the onion fine."

They may be humble, but members of the lily family are some of the most powerful aphrodisiacs and wonder drugs on the planet. Whether your tastes run toward garlic, onions, shallots, leeks, or asparagus, these versatile vegetables will help bring good health and healthy sex.

Plus, they deter evil! You can't get that from a watermelon.

The cooking couple's LovabLe LiLies and Amorous ALLiums menu for Amour

{ Ajo BLanco con uvas }
(GarLic and ALmond soup with Grapes)

This wonderful garlicky Spanish soup makes a refreshing first course, requires no cooking, and will really raise your nitric oxide levels. For a light meal, serve with gorgonzola or goat cheese and toasted rustic bread spread with fig jam.

4 ounces blanched almonds

1 ounce pine nuts

5 garlic cloves, peeled

½ cup soft, white bread crumbs

3 cups ice water

4 tablespoons olive oil

2 tablespoons red wine or sherry vinegar

1 teaspoon salt

6 ounces seedless grapes

1. In a food processor chop almonds, pine nuts, and garlic. (Do not over-process or oil will separate from nuts.) Add bread crumbs and 1 cup ice water and process until mixture resembles a thin paste. With processor running, carefully add olive oil, vinegar, and salt.

2. Pour mixture into a bowl or soup tureen, mix in remaining 2 cups ice water. Refrigerate soup until ready to serve.

3. To serve, ladle soup into bowls and add grapes on top.

Serves 6

{ Soupe a' L'oignon gratinée }
(French onion soup)

The next time you and your lover are snowbound with only a few pantry staples, whip up a batch of *Soupe a' l'oignon gratinée* (onion soup). Open a bottle of red wine and enjoy this gooey treat. According to legend, this soup was invented one evening by a hungry King Louis XV because his hunting lodge pantry contained only onions, butter, and champagne. The port adds flavor and color, but it is optional.

2 tablespoons butter

1 tablespoon olive oil

5 large onions, thinly sliced

1 cup dry white wine

½ cup port or brandy

6 cups chicken stock or canned low-sodium beef or chicken broth

1 teaspoon sugar

4 thick slices French bread, toasted

¾ cup grated Gruyère cheese

1. In a large stock pot, heat butter and oil over medium heat. Add the onions, lower heat, and cook uncovered, stirring occasionally, until onions are soft, brown, and caramelized, about 30 minutes.

2. Add the wine and brandy or port, bring to a boil and cook until reduced by half, about 5 minutes. Add stock and sugar and bring to a boil. Reduce heat and simmer the soup, partially covered, for 30 minutes. Add salt and pepper to taste. (Soup can be made up to this point and refrigerated.)

3. To serve, ladle hot soup into oven-safe bowls, top with French bread and grated Gruyère cheese, and place under broiler until cheese melts.

Serves 4

{ Easy GarLic Dressing }

Pour on salads or use as an allium marinade for chicken or fish.

4 garlic cloves, minced

$\frac{1}{2}$ teaspoon salt

$\frac{1}{2}$ teaspoon freshly ground black pepper

$\frac{1}{2}$ cup olive oil

$\frac{1}{3}$ cup balsamic vinegar

Place all ingredients in an air-tight container and shake well to combine.

{ Arabic Egg Mash }
(scrambLed Eggs with onion and Aphro spices)

According to Sheikh Nefzaoui, "He who peels onions, puts them into a saucepan with condiments and aromatic substances, and fries the mixture with oil and yolks of eggs, will acquire a surpassing and invaluable vigor for the coitus, if he will partake of this dish for several days." So what are you waiting for?

4 eggs

Pinch of Kosher salt

1 tablespoon butter

2 large onions, peeled and thinly sliced

$\frac{1}{2}$ teaspoon curry powder

$\frac{1}{4}$ teaspoon cardamom

1 tablespoon chopped fresh cilantro for garnish

1. In a small bowl, whisk together eggs and salt.
2. Melt butter in a large nonstick skillet over medium-low heat. Add onions and sauté until soft, about 10 minutes.
3. Add the curry powder and cardamom to the skillet, and cook for about 30 seconds. Add the eggs and cook, slowly stirring, until eggs are set, 2 to 3 minutes.
4. Place eggs on plates, sprinkle with chopped cilantro, and serve with warm pita bread, melted butter, and honey.

Serves 2

{ Roasted Figs and onions }

This recipe works well as a side dish with roasted meat or poultry or as an appetizer served with goat cheese and toasted French bread.

2 red onions, peeled and cut in quarters

2 tablespoons olive oil

Salt and freshly ground black pepper to taste

4 fresh figs

1 tablespoon balsamic vinegar

2 tablespoon fresh herbs, finely chopped

2 tablespoons pine nuts

1. Preheat oven to 350° F.
2. Toss onions with olive oil, salt, and pepper. Place onions in a roasting pan and cook, stirring occasionally, in preheated oven for 30 minutes.
3. Add figs and cook, basting occasionally, for another 15 minutes.
4. Gently toss onions and figs with herbs and balsamic vinegar. Serve topped with pine nuts.

Serves 2 as an appetizer or side dish

{ Aphro chicken }
(chicken with 40 cloves of garlic)

This is based on James Beard's simple recipe from the French region of Provence. For a complete meal, serve with an earthy red wine such as Syrah, a simple salad, and French bread, using the roasted garlic as a spread.

1 whole frying chicken, about 3 to 4 pounds, or 4 thigh quarters with leg

Coarse salt and freshly ground black pepper to taste

40 large garlic cloves, separated and unpeeled

2 medium onions, coarsely chopped

2 stalks celery, chopped

½ cup fresh, mixed herbs, chopped

2 tablespoons olive oil

⅓ cup dry white wine or vermouth

1. Preheat oven to 375° F.

2. Season the chicken (both inside and out, if it is a whole chicken) with salt and pepper.

3. If using thighs and legs, place all ingredients in a large Dutch oven or other deep, heavy pot with a cover and combine well. If using a whole chicken, tuck 3 tablespoons of herbs and about a dozen garlic cloves inside cavity, place bird on top of onions and celery, scatter remaining garlic cloves around pan, and pour olive oil and wine over top of chicken.

4. Cover pot and seal tightly with aluminum foil so no steam escapes. Bake for 1½ hours.

Serves 4

{ Asparagus-stuffed steak }

This elegant dish can be prepared several hours in advance and roasted while you and your guest . . .

1 (3½- to 4-pound) flank steak, approximately 1 inch thick

3 tablespoons horseradish mustard

4 garlic cloves, minced

1 pound fresh asparagus, trimmed and peeled

1. Preheat over to 350° F. Using a large, sharp knife, butterfly the steak by slicing through the meat horizontally without cutting all the way through, so that the two halves can be opened like a book or butterfly. Open the meat and spread with the mustard and sprinkle with garlic. Place asparagus spears in a single row over the mustard and garlic. Roll meat tightly and tie with kitchen twine.

2. Roast meat in preheated oven for 1 hour. Let meat rest for 10 minutes. Slice into rounds, and serve.

Serves 4 and makes great leftovers

{ Lily Melange }
(Asparagus with onions and Garlic)

Another aphrodisiac triple-header. This terrific Italian side dish could be called "Amore in the Produce Market."

1½ pounds asparagus

2 medium sweet onions, such as Vidalia, minced

½ cup extra-virgin olive oil

¼ cup lemon juice

2 garlic cloves, minced

2 teaspoons lemon zest

2 medium tomatoes or 1 red pepper, diced

Salt and freshly ground black pepper to taste

1. Steam asparagus until tender and bright green, about 5 minutes. Submerge spears in ice water to stop cooking process. Drain and pat dry with paper towels.
2. Combine remaining ingredients, toss with cooked asparagus, and serve immediately.

Serves 4

8

Enticing Herbs and seductive spices

*I have perfumed my bed with myrrh, aloes, and cinnamon.
Come, let us take our fill of love until morning, let us solace our-
selves with love.*

—Proverbs 7:17-18

In the Middle Ages, spices were worth their weight in gold, and herbs were highly valued for their medicinal and magical powers. Frankincense and myrrh, cinnamon, cardamom, and ginger were the designer drugs of the day. Fortunes were made and lost, wars were fought, and lives were sacrificed all in the name of herbs and spices. On the bones of many, and the stems, buds, flowers, and roots of these delicate delicacies, the first global commodity was born.

Erotic Aromatherapy

The botanicals craved centuries ago were and still are sought after for their sexually stimulating effects. In India and China, where many of these seductively scented plants originated, people understood the power of aromatherapy and realized that herbs and spices could enhance sexual vitality and provide a whiff of postcoital rejuvenation. The *Ananga Ranga,* the Arabic love manual, teaches that spices can help you "ascend the throne of love and gratify each other's desires."

The author of the *Kama Sutra,* India's Scripture of Love, un-

sensual scents

Essential oils, the concentrated essence of various flowers, fruits, herbs, spices, and plants, are an easy way to ignite passion, increase energy, and reduce stress. You can use a single oil, buy a combination of oils that have been blended for a specific purpose, or make your own personal blend to perfume your body or environment.

Sexy essential oils include cinnamon, cardamom, pepper, sandalwood, musk, patchouli, ylang ylang, jasmine, rose, clary, sage, and neroli. We can't predict which ones will turn you and your lover on, so experiment together and note each other's reactions. To get started, here are several ways to incorporate essential oils into your love life.

- In the bath—Add 3 to 5 drops directly to the water, place 1 drop on a loofah sponge, or mix 10 drops with 2 ounces of liquid soap.
- For a massage—Mix 15 drops with 2 ounces of neutral oil such as canola, almond, or olive.
- In the bedroom—Place 5 to 15 drops of essential oil in a lamp ring or aromatherapy lamp (both of which are available in natural food stores) or place 10 drops in 1 quart of water and use the mixture to mist the air.
- For your dresser drawers—Place 2 drops of essential oil on a piece of felt and use to keep you and your clothes smelling fabulous.
- For your hair—Mix 4 drops essential oil with an ounce of shampoo or conditioner, or place 2 drops on hair brush bristles before use.

derstood the connection between body odor and sexual excitation. Indian women used saffron, musk, amber, and sandalwood to encourage sexual excitement and create an attractive atmosphere.

Today, science is confirming what our ancestors knew all along: that certain scents are a sexual turn on. The smell of pumpkin pie spice (which is a combination of cinnamon, ginger, and clove) combined with lavender increases penile blood flow in men by an average of 40 percent, according to the Smell and Taste Treatment and Research Foundation.

But why?

Our sense of smell is our most primitive sense. The nerve endings in the nose are closely connected to the old mammalian center of the brain, the limbic system, which is the switchboard for our emotions, moods, and basic instincts—including sexual desire. This is the part of the brain that also picks up pheromones, molecules released into the air by one animal that attract another animal of the same species, usually of the opposite sex.

The word *spice* comes from the Latin word *species,* and originally meant a type of merchandise. Spices were small and light, yet valuable, making them an ideal commodity for trade, and were even used as currency. Spices were prized as one of the few ways to preserve and make food taste better. The growing merchant class of the Middle Ages demonstrated their culinary sophistication and wealth with spices. Meanwhile, merchants in the East wanted gold and silver, and were happy to trade their spices for these precious metals. Spices were also highly prized for their medicinal and aphrodisiacal properties.

The demand and the cost of obtaining spices made them expensive, particularly for European countries that had to import them from as far as halfway around the world. (This was very tough to do back when the earth was flat.) The dangerous journey to obtain spices could take years, and every middleman along the way needed to get his cut. By the time a pound of pepper or vanilla reached the West, its price could have increased by as much as fortyfold.

The stakes were so high that men were willing to risk everything for a few pounds of pepper, quintals of mace, or sticks of cinnamon. In 1540, a Spanish explorer named Francisco Pizarro took 2,000 men to search for a mythical cinnamon forest purportedly located in uncharted regions of South America. The party traveled for months through constant rain, across paths that were too narrow for their horses, while occasionally stopping to torture natives along the way for information. Only eighty of Pizarro's men survived.

To a large extent, the struggle for spices paralleled the struggle for empires. In 1492, the New World was discovered by accident. All Columbus was trying to do was find a faster route to the East for spices when he bumped into the New World. ("Ah, what the hell, guys. We're here, so we might as well conquer it.")

In the words of Sir Walter Raleigh, "The discovery of the new Western World followed, as an incidental consequence, from the long struggle of the nations of Europe for commercial supremacy and control of the traffic with the East. In all these dreams of the politicians and merchants, sailors and geographers, who pushed back the limits of the unknown world, there is the same glitter of gold and precious stones, the same odor of far-fetched spices."

Prior to the Middle Ages, the profits from trading spices made Italian city-states like Florence, Genoa, and Venice wealthy and

Herbs and spices, understanding the difference

Although some herbal plants yield a spice—cilantro produces the spice coriander—and both herbs and spices are used as flavorings and aphrodisiacs, there is a big difference between them.

Spices are generally defined as the dried parts (roots, bulbs, bark, buds, fruit, seeds, or leaves) of various pungent plants used in cooking to season or flavor food. They usually grow in warm tropical or subtropical regions and are cultivated for their aromatic properties.

Herbs are the fragrant leaves (and sometimes stems) of green plants that do not grow larger like trees or shrubs, but wither at the end of the season. (The word *herb* comes from the Latin *herba,* which means a grass or other green plant.) They usually grow in temperate regions and are preferably used fresh.

powerful. At the start of the fifteenth century, nation-states took up the spice cause, spending huge sums and even setting up navigation schools to find better spice routes. In the early 1400s, Prince Henry the Navigator of Portugal started organizing overseas explorations because the Ottoman Empire was making travel via the traditional land routes difficult. He supported sailors, mapmakers, astronomers, and shipbuilders in hopes of finding a way around Africa to the Orient.

Herbal Enticements

Better is a dinner of herbs where love is than a fatted ox and hatred with it.

–Proverbs 15:17

Herbs, particularly when fresh and used with abandon, are a wonderful way to accent and enhance the flavor of foods and awaken a slumbering libido. In *A Midsummer Night's Dream,* Shakespeare acknowledged the passionate power of herbs when he wrote, "powerful herb, the juice of which on sleeping eyelids laid will make man or woman madly dote upon the next live creature that it sees."

Many herbs also have valuable healing properties that can help reverse medical problems such as fatigue, stress, and urinary tract and vaginal infections that interfere with sexual vitality. Other herbs, such as caraway seeds, which were chewed to promote the desire to procreate, can help increase libido, improve sexual performance, and even intensify sexual pleasure. Here are some of our favorite aphrodisiacal herbs.

HOLY BASIL

Woman is like a fruit which will only yield its fragrance when rubbed by the hands. Take, for example, the basil; unless it be warmed by the fingers it emits no perfume.

–Sheikh Nefzaoui, *The Perfumed Garden*

It's hard to believe that simple basil, which grows easily on a windowsill, was considered sacred in India where it originated, was named for royalty in Greece, and was believed to produce and summon serpents and scorpions. (The herb was originally named "basilik," for a mythical fire-breathing serpent.) Used in voodoo love ceremonies in Haiti, foods flavored with basil are believed to help lovers reunite after a fight.

Hindu men claim basil resembles female genitals, and in Romania, when a man accepts basil from his love it means he is engaged. Basil can also help you out once you are hitched. Latin women sprinkle dried basil leaves on their bodies to stop their husbands from sleeping around.

Basil's erotic, unique licoricey flavor can perk up a variety of dishes. The main ingredient in pesto and the French soup garnish *pistou,* basil pairs beautifully with tomatoes and works wonders in salads, pasta dishes, pizza, vegetable soups, curries, and Asian stir-fries. Just make sure to treat it tenderly. While basil plants are hearty, it's best to gently tear the leaves. Cutting basil bruises the leaves, which discolors them and decreases flavor.

PARSLEY, MR. POPULAR

The most popular culinary herb and nature's breath freshener, parsley is high in histidine, an amino acid that the body converts to histamine, a molecule that regulates ejaculation and orgasm. Studies conducted by Dr. Carl Pfeiffer, author of *Mental and Ele-*

Benefits Beyond the Bedroom

Not only will culinary herbs and spices spice up your love life, eating them on a regular basis can also make you healthier by boosting the immune system and decreasing your risk of cardiovascular disease and hypertension.

Sprinkling cinnamon, thyme, tarragon, and cumin on meat killed up to 80 percent of bacteria and other microbes, preventing food poisoning, according to two researchers from Cornell University. Garlic, onions, allspice, and oregano destroyed almost 100 percent of the microscopic invaders. That's one reason why, in hot climates where food-borne illness is a potential hazard, people use a tremendous amount of herbs and spices in their food.

mental Nutrients: A Physician's Guide to Nutrition and Health Care, have shown that frigidity can be reversed by supplementing the diet with the amino acid L-histidine. Histidine also works as a vasodilator, making blood flow to the sex organs easier, and it may inhibit tumor growth.

Parsley is rich in vitamins A and C, potassium, and iron, and also contains three phytochemicals: apiole, apiin, and pinene, which help improve digestion, eliminate bloating, and decrease blood pressure. Just don't eat too much if you are pregnant. In large amounts, parsley can cause uterine contractions.

In parts of England, parsley wine is consumed as an aphrodisiac, and the phrase "curly parsley" was once used as British slang for "pubic hair." Parsley symbolizes new beginnings and, according to folklore, sowing parsley seeds is also believed to enhance fertility.

The French believe parsley sparks the libido, an idea that comes from the Greek physician Dioscorides, who said parsley "provokes venery and bodily lust." In Spain, parsley is fed to sheep to bring them into heat. Romans believed eating parsley would prevent them from getting drunk. (How about just not drinking so much? Perhaps we should call it the "falling down" of the Roman Empire.) The custom of garnishing a plate with parsley was first used to protect food from evil and increase wealth.

Flat-leaf parsley is stronger than curly parsley and works in most savory dishes. It harmonizes well with other herbs and gives a clean, fresh flavor to any recipe it touches, from salads, to soups and fish, to vegetable dishes.

Aphrodite's crown is in mint condition

The smell of mint does stir up the minde and the taste to a greedy desire of meat.

–John Gerard,
English botanist (1545-1612)

If you want to leave your lover fresh, unwilted, and yearning for more sex after a dose of passion, share a sprig or two of mint. According to the noted Swiss psychiatrist and father of the collective unconscious, Carl Gustav Jung, in ancient times mint, which is ruled by the planet Venus, was called "Aphrodite's crown."

One of the best-known oils used for aromatherapy, mint stimulates the central hippocampus, the part of the brain responsible for consolidating memories into permanent storage. Mint's seductive allure is practically ingrained in our psyches.

A beautiful nymph named Minthe, who also was the daughter of Ceres (goddess of agriculture), was messing with Pluto, god of the underworld, behind his wife, Persephone's, back. (Most mints are very promiscuous, happily mating with other plants in the garden to form new hybrids.) When she found out about the affair, jealous Persephone turned Minthe into a plant. (Do *not* piss off goddesses. Even minor ones.) While Pluto could not reverse the spell, he could modify it so that the more Minthe was stepped on the sweeter she smelled. Despite the transformation, Pluto still found Minthe, especially her aroma, irresistible.

In honor of Minthe, Greek brides include mint in their bridal wreath. The Greek philosopher Aristotle knew peppermint was an aphrodisiac when he prohibited Alexander the Great's soldiers from eating it because he wanted them to make war, not love. The Romans brought mint to England, where, like many other herbs, it was cultivated in monastery gardens during the Middle Ages.

Mint is also valuable in treating indigestion, congestion, insomnia, and nausea. (A study published in the *Journal of Advanced Nursing* detailed mint's success in stopping postoperative nausea.) Crushed mint leaves can also be placed on the forehead as a headache remedy, or rubbed on the skin to relieve the itch of insect bites. Try refreshing your lover by rubbing his or her sore muscles and aching feet with a little mint-scented massage oil.

Pliny, who said, "Mint exhilarates the mind and stimulates the brain" recommended that scholars wear mint wreaths to aid their concentration, and sniffing mint may help improve memory.

There are hundreds of varieties of mint, all of which are part of the *Mentha* family. Chocolate mint smells like a peppermint patty, and can be crushed and used to flavor coffee or warm milk. There are also many types of fruit mints, including grapefruit, pineapple, apple, and lime, as well as ginger, which can be added to iced tea or juice or used as a garnish for fruit salad.

Spearmint is most commonly used fresh and dried for cooking. It is often incorporated into jams, jellies, and sauces that accompany meat, fish, and vegetable dishes, especially lamb, and it is also used to garnish fruit drinks. Mint is used to flavor candy, gum, toothpaste, and condoms.

In the Arab world, mint tea is popular, and fresh mint leaves are added to bulgur wheat (to make tabbouleh) and yogurt. To

Anyone for a Mint Julep?

Every year on Derby Day, the first Saturday in May, Churchill Downs serves 80,000 mint juleps. But you don't have to wait for the Kentucky Derby or watch several thousand pounds of horse flesh run around a track with midgets on their backs whipping them (sounds like a David Lynch movie) to enjoy a mint julep. All you need are a hot day, fresh mint, sugar, ice, and bourbon and you're ready for a refreshing afternoon pick-me-up.

The mint julep's ancestor was a refreshing Arabic drink made with water and rose petals called a julab. When the julab was introduced to the Mediterranean, people replaced the rose petals with mint. In the nineteenth century, whiskey was added to the drink, which quickly became popular with American farmers, who drank juleps in the morning. Like farmers, horse trainers also rise at the crack of dawn, and began jump-starting their day with juleps. (How did these people get anything done?) The julep became associated with horse races, and gradually made the transition from morning drink to afternoon cocktail.

While the official mint julep of the Kentucky Derby calls for making mint syrup ahead of time, we've devised a quicker version so you can be sitting and sipping your juleps by post time. (That's 5:30 P.M. on Derby Day.) Although we're not conservative by nature, we do believe that A.M. imbibing does cut into general productivity.

{ Mint Julep }

3 sprigs fresh mint

1 teaspoon superfine sugar

2 ounces Kentucky bourbon (Bourbon is whiskey that contains
at least 51 percent corn mash. While bourbon can come
from anywhere, Kentucky bourbon must come from
Kentucky.)

Bruise (crush) the leaves from two sprigs of mint, and add to a small glass, along with the sugar and 1 tablespoon of water. Add the bourbon, stir, and strain into a Collins glass filled with crushed or shaved ice. Stir and serve garnished with an additional sprig of mint.

Makes 1 drink

{ MOJITO }

If you want to turn your mate into a red-hot Latin lover, try a mojito. This stimulating, light-rum-based, mint-spiked Cuban cocktail is perfect for a summer night of sipping and samba.

4 fresh mint leaves, plus one whole sprig for garnish

Dash simple syrup*

1½ ounces rum

Club soda

In a Collins glass, muddle (crush) mint leaves and add a dash of simple syrup. Fill glass with ice. Add rum, top with club soda, and garnish with mint sprig.

Makes 1 drink

*To make simple syrup, mix one part water with 2 parts sugar. Heat mixture until sugar dissolves. Cool and store in a plastic squeeze bottle in the refrigerator.

test the aphrodisiacal properties of mint, brew up a batch of Moroccan-style mint tea at home. In a teapot, steep several sprigs of spearmint with green tea and boiling water. Sweeten with sugar or honey. If you really want to be authentic, pour the tea into a tall narrow glass from several feet above the table, and serve with *qa'b el-ghazal* ("horns of the doe"), orange-flavored crescent pastries filled with almond paste.

Herb Tips

As a flavor accent and aphrodisiac, there is no substitute for fresh herbs, which readily release their aromatic essential oils when rubbed, steeped, or cooked. At one time, only parsley was readily available in grocery stores, but fortunately, today hot house cultivation has made a variety of fresh herbs available all year long. Many are also easy to grow. Purchase potted herbs in a garden store or nursery, place them either outside (in warm weather), or on your windowsill, and snip whenever needed.

Once gathered, fresh herbs perish in about 3 to 4 days. To keep them fresh, place stem end of herbs in a little water (like you would for flowers) and store in the refrigerator.

You can also wrap fresh herbs in a damp paper towel and place them in a plastic bag. Or they can be washed in cold water, blanched, dried completely, and frozen in small airtight bags.

Fresh herbs should be minced or chopped right before use and added to hot foods, except when making stock, when they should be added at the last minute. For an unusual and tasty centerpiece, wash the herbs, place in water, and allow diners to snip herbs and sprinkle on their food as they eat.

Dried herbs (under ideal conditions) will keep for up to six months, stored in a cool, dry place. To bring out the most flavor in dried herbs, steep them for about 15 minutes in a warm liquid such as melted butter, stock, or water. If a recipe calls for fresh herbs and you have only dried (or vice versa) you can substitute 1 teaspoon of loosely packed dried herbs for 2 teaspoons fresh chopped herbs.

Another way to enjoy herbs all year long is to use herb-flavored oils, vinegars, salts, mustards, and sauces either in recipes or as condiments.

Damiana, Another Aphrodisiac from the Aztecs

As if chocolate, chiles, avocados, and vanilla weren't enough, the Aztecs are also responsible for introducing the world to the herb damiana (a.k.a. *Turnera aphrodosoaca*), which they used as an aphrodisiac. Available in most health food stores, today both men and women throughout the world use the herb, a shrub that grows in Mexico, Central and South America, and the West Indies, to improve sexual function.

Damiana strengthens the genitourinary and renal tracts, boosting the health of the reproductive system, and can create a tingling sensation in the genitals. It has been used as an aphrodisiac in the United States for about a century to reverse sterility and impotence and increase overall vitality. According to David Hoffman, author of *The New Holistic Herbal,* "The pharmacology of the plant suggests that the alkaloids could have testosterone-like actions."

Like the herb kava, damiana is also a nerve stimulant that promotes feelings of well-being and reduces anxiety, both of which can make you feel more open sexually. However, unlike kava, damiana has many more unpleasant and potentially dangerous side effects that include heart palpitations and vomiting, and may interact badly with prescription medications, particularly those for high blood pressure and depression. Take this herb only under the supervision of a physician who has experience working with damiana.

Yohimbe

Years before Viagra hit medicine cabinets across the country, a drug made from yohimbe bark called Yohimbine was approved by the Food and Drug Administration (FDA) for the treatment of male sexual dysfunction. Dubbed "herbal Viagra" by the newsletter *Environmental Nutrition,* yohimbe bark comes from the yohimbe tree, a native of West Africa, where it has been used to increase the libido for hundreds of years. Discovered as an aphrodisiac by Europeans about seventy years ago, today yohimbe bark is sold in health food stores across the country as an herbal supplement, and can be combined with other herbs in sex-enhancing formulas.

Yohimbine, the active chemical in yohimbe bark, works by blocking nerves that constrict blood vessels. This helps blood vessels dilate, increasing blood flow to the penis, thus improving erections. A Stanford University study found that subjects taking yohimbe bark extract experienced nearly a 100 percent increase in sexual desire in less than one hour.

Along with boosting sexual performance and libido, the herb also appears to fight the blues by increasing levels of mood-enhancing neurotransmitters, such as serotonin, in the brain.

Although yohimbe bark is widely available in health food stores and on the Internet, it does have a number of unpleasant side effects, including vomiting, nausea, anxiety, and increased blood pressure, and should be used under the supervision of a physician who has experience with the herb yohimbe bark or the drug Yohimbine.

spicing up Romance

Used in love potions and as stimulants, offered to fertility gods, applied topically to enlarge the penis, and sprinkled on wedding beds to increase passion, spices have a long history as aphrodisiacs. Hindu and Arabic cultures, recognizing that these substances could stimulate sexual activity, trained cooks in the art of preparing and using aphrodisiacal spices. One Persian recipe calls for placing cloves, cinnamon, and cardamom in a jar, then reciting a chapter of the Koran backward. Add rose water, one of your husband's shirts, and a piece of parchment inscribed with your husband's name and the names of four angels, and bring the mixture to a boil over a fire.

Europeans were also keen on using spices as aphrodisiacs. In the fifteenth century, one German ruler had all his lovers rubbed with spices so that he could pick the woman who most suited his flavor craving of the moment. ("I'll take the blond with the cinnamon streaks, and two redheads with ginger highlights.") And during the reign of Louis XIV the dependably decadent French went overboard (as usual), rubbing their bodies with cinnamon and spiking their food with generous amounts of spices. *Fini,* already!

So, if you want to start spicing up your love life (with or without the full body rub), read on.

pepper, the king of spices

Looking to pump up Mr. Happy, boys? Pepper just might do the trick. *The Perfumed Garden* recommends making a powder from pepper, lavender, galanga (also called Siamese ginger), and musk, mixing it with honey and preserved ginger, and vigorously rubbing the mixture over your penis. Your penis "will then grow large and brawny and afford the woman a marvelous feeling of voluptuousness." The Chinese penis prescription calls for boiling pimento and pepper together with the herb mallow, and mixing with a rice flour to make a poultice that can be applied topically to stimulate the penis.

To increase their sexual desire and ability to copulate frequently, ancient Greek lovers mixed pepper with nettle seeds and used it as a condiment. Pepper is also recommended in the *Kama Sutra:* "If a man anoints his penis with datura, black pepper, and long pepper (a spice in the same family as black pepper that was used extensively in ancient and medieval times), crushed and mixed with honey, its use will allow him to bewitch and subjugate his partners." Hey, and if subjugation isn't enough and you still can't get it up, the *Kama Sutra* suggests: "Mix garlic root with

Other Aphrodisiacs in the Pepper Family

Your head is affected most pleasantly. Thoughts come cleanly. You feel friendly . . . never cross . . . You cannot hate with kava in you.

–Tom Harrison, author, *Savage Civilization*

• In the Polynesian Islands, *Piper methysticum* (which means "intoxicating pepper" and is also known as kava kava) has been used for religious rituals and as an aphrodisiac and medicine for at least 3,000 years. Pacific Island natives blend chewed or pounded kava root with coconut milk and allow the mixture to ferment. When ingested, it produces a sense of euphoria and relaxation and sometimes a tingling in the genitals. Kava is also rubbed directly on the clitoris prior to oral sex.

Kava is taken today to decrease anxiety, relieve pain, and promote relaxation. The relaxed state, sense of euphoria, and sharpening of the senses kava produces contribute to its aphrodisiacal effect. Kava is also used to treat a variety of disorders of the genitourinary tract that can interfere with your sex life including vaginitis, cystitis, prostitis, gonorrhea, and menstrual cramps.

Kava should be used in moderation. Overuse can cause a variety of side effects including scaly skin and shortness of breath, all of which are reversible when you stop taking it. Based on anti-anxiety studies, the recommended daily dose is 70 to 210 milligrams of kavalactones. (Kavalactone is the active ingredient in kava.) Pregnant or nursing women and people being treated for depression should not take kava. You should not mix kava with alcohol, sedatives, or tranquilizers.

• The Chinese drank an infusion made from cubeb pepper leaves (a fragrant, large pepper, *Piper cubeba*, native to Indonesia and sometimes called Java pepper) to increase sexual desire, strengthen and enlarge the penis, and to prevent gonorrhea.

•The Peruvian Indians use matico leaves as an aphrodisiac. Matico, *Piper angustifolium,* grows in the tropical regions of the Americas and was named for a Spanish soldier who accidentally discovered that the leaves helped stop bleeding when he was wounded in Peru.

white pepper and licorice. When drunk with sugared milk, it enhances virility." Another common Indian aphrodisiac, which doubles as a nerve tonic, is mixing six crushed black peppercorns with four crushed almonds and a glass of milk, and drinking it daily.

Now you know why pepper is the most popular spice in the world.

Today, a powerful essential oil made from black pepper is frequently combined with other sexy scents such as ylang ylang and patchouli and added to soaps, perfumes, and massage oils to provide a warm, earthy, erotic aroma. Black pepper essential oil is sharp and spicy, and is used in aromatherapy to stimulate and strengthen the nerves, increase stamina, and warm the heart. Its scent is also believed to dilate blood vessels, improve circulation, and stimulate the appetite. As you will learn later in our chapter "The Cooking Couple's Best Sex Diet," increasing circulation and improving stamina play major roles in improving sexual vitality.

Unlike chile peppers, the spice pepper gets its heat from the volatile oils peperine, chavicine, peperidine, and piperettine. It improves the appetite by increasing salivation and the flow of gastric juices and helps create a feeling of fullness. Hey, it's a diet aid and an aphrodisiac!

All pepper—black, green, and white—comes from the berry of the *Piper nigrum* plant, a native of India. Pepper berries grow on a vine in grape-like clusters, and are picked when they are green and then spread out in the sun for several days to dry, shrink, and turn into the hard, black spice commonly referred to as black pepper. Green peppercorns are picked several weeks before black ones and tend to be milder. Berries used to make white pepper ripen longer on the vine and are soaked in water after harvest to remove the outer coating.

There are many types of black pepper, which are named for the region in which they are grown and, like tea and chile peppers, vary in terms of flavor and heat. Some of the more interesting varieties include Malabar (a small, spicy pepper with citrus notes); Tellicherry (a larger, sweeter pepper with a fruity flavor), usually from India; Sarawak (a mild, earthy pepper), usually from Malaysia; and Lampong (a hotter pepper with a fruity flavor), usually from Indonesia.

One of the earliest spices known to mankind, pepper was highly valued by the Egyptians, Greeks, and Romans. The Roman scholar Pliny complained about its price, and Alaric, king of the Visigoths, demanded 3,000 pounds of pepper as part of a ransom for Rome. (He settled for three virgins, a bottle of Jägermeister, and two fourth-row tickets to a Springsteen concert at the Coliseum.)

After the fall of the Roman Empire, pepper remained an extremely important commodity. It was a key element in the spice trade between Europe and India and was referenced in English records as far back as A.D. 978. Pepper was so precious in medieval Europe that workers unloading shipments of pepper dressed in clothing without pockets to thwart theft, much as workers mining diamonds do today. It was used as currency, included in bridal dowries, and employed to bribe judges.

There was even an English pepper guild called the Pepperers, who in 1328 registered their name as Grossari, which is where the word grocer comes from.

cinnamon

You know, I really don't think I need buns of steel. I'd be happy with buns of cinnamon.

—ELLen DeGeneres

One of the oldest spices known, cinnamon has been a popular aphrodisiac and ingredient in love potions for centuries. The pungent, inviting spice works particularly well when combined with chocolate (which is common in Mexico) and apples. The Queen of Sheba used cinnamon to charm King Solomon, and Nero burned a year's worth of the spice in remorse after he murdered his wife. (See, he really did care.)

The sweet, spicy aroma of cinnamon oil is used to help reverse impotence, improve mood, and fight fatigue. Personally we feel the warm, inviting smell of freshly baked cinnamon buns (another scientifically proven aphrodisiac from the Smell and Taste Treatment and Research Foundation) is a great excuse to cuddle in bed on a frosty morning. Serve those buns with Turkish coffee

simple ways to use cinnamon

Here are a few ways to use cinnamon as a love food:
- Chew on sticks of cinnamon or cassia as you think about your lover.
- Make heart-shaped cinnamon toast. Using a cookie cutter, cut white bread into the shape of a heart. Spread bread with butter, sprinkle with cinnamon sugar, and toast. Or top heart-shaped French toast with cinnamon sugar.
- To arouse the woman in your life, sprinkle cinnamon on egg dishes.
- Garnish coffee or hot chocolate with a cinnamon stick.
- Toast your love with a cinnamon-flavored cocktail.

cinnamon at the bar

Cinnamon also works its wonders in a variety of cocktails and in coffee drinks. Here are some ideas to get you started.

{ Indian summer }

1 cup apple cider
Cinnamon
2 ounces apple schnapps
1 cinnamon stick
Gently warm cider. Dampen the rim of a sour glass and dip it in cinnamon. Pour schnapps into the glass and top off with warmed cider. Garnish with a cinnamon stick.

{ Fireball }

2 ounces cinnamon schnapps
Dash Tabasco
Fill a shot glass with cinnamon schnapps. Top with Tabasco and shoot.

{ Granny's Apple cinnamon shotgun }

3 Granny Smith apples (or any tart apple)
2 cinnamon sticks
1 (750 ml) bottle vodka
Cut the apples into quarters, remove cores, but do not peel. Place apples in a large jar. Add cinnamon sticks and vodka. Let sit at room temperature for 3 to 4 days. Store in the refrigerator or freezer and use within 2 to 3 weeks. Serve ice cold alone (or on the rocks if you prefer) or with a shot of cinnamon schnapps garnished with a cinnamon stick.

(a combination of strong coffee with aphrodisiacs including cinnamon, cardamom, cloves, and nutmeg) and you're in for a day of fun.

Today, two ounces of powdered cinnamon costs about $2.79. Two thousand years ago, cinnamon was worth fifteen times its weight in silver and was a major player in the spice trade. Between the twelfth and fourteenth centuries, Arabic traders who first brought the spice to the West kept the origins of cinnamon a secret and shrouded it in mystery. (According to stories fabricated by traders, cinnamon came from the nests of the Phoenix or from the blood of fighting dragons and elephants.)

Finding cinnamon was one of the goals of explorers in the fifteenth and sixteenth centuries. The Portuguese found it in 1505 on the island of Ceylon, which was taken over by the Dutch in 1636. The island was then conquered by the French and later by the British. Trading lives for cinnamon during the spice wars was considered a sound investment.

Most cinnamon sold in the United States is actually cassia bark (also called Chinese cinnamon) or a combination of cassia and real cinnamon. Although a bit more pungent, cassia is virtually identical to real cinnamon both in terms of taste and aphrodisiacal powers. Cinnamon can be used in both sweet and savory dishes, particularly baked goods, fruit compote, and marinades for meat and poultry, as well as in Middle Eastern meat stews such as tangine.

cilantro and its seed, coriander

The medieval philosopher and occultist Albertus Magnus believed that coriander, along with the soothing herb valerian and violets, produced love when gathered when the moon was almost new. (Violets and cilantro were also an early American folk remedy for hangovers.) In *A Thousand and One Tales of the Arabian Nights,* liquor spiked with coriander is consumed as an aphrodisiac. During the Han dynasty (207 B.C.-A.D. 200), coriander was used as an aphrodisiac, and the Chinese also used it for immortality. (We are a bit dubious about this immortality stuff.)

While coriander and cilantro are associated with Asian, Mexican, and Indian food (the seeds are standard in the curry spice mix garam masala) the plant actually hails from the Mediterranean where, in its wild form, it was consumed during the Bronze Age. The Romans used coriander and cilantro as a food and medicine and took the plant with them as they conquered the ancient world. Coriander mixed with vinegar was used as an early meat tenderizer and preservative. Sugar-coated coriander seeds were the original sugarplums enjoyed by children during Christmas. Today, the seeds are used in Belgian specialty beers such as Hoegaarden, and medicinally to freshen the breath and settle the stomach.

Like anchovies and garlic, most people are either passionate about the herb cilantro and its offspring coriander, or they hate it. Both have a powerful smell. Cilantro, which is also known as Chinese parsley, has a strong, almost citrusy flavor sometimes described as soapy. Coriander, whose name comes from the Greek word for bed bug, *koris,* has a foul smell when freshly picked that becomes intense, sweet, and spicy as it ripens.

Before you use coriander or cilantro as a love food, we recommend that you taste and experiment with the seasonings to see if you and your partner like them. Try using fresh cilantro as a garnish instead of parsley, or sprinkle the chopped herb on Latin and Asian dishes. Ground coriander seed can be used to flavor stews and curries, and it can be added to sweet baked goods. To enhance the libido, add a pinch of ground coriander seeds to a bottle of red or white wine and let the mixture steep for a week, shaking every few days. Strain out the seeds and drink.

Cardamom: The Queen of Spices

Since being featured in *Tales of the Arabian Nights*, people have been dipping into cardamom, a member of the ginger family, to enhance sexual vitality. The Arabic love text *The Perfumed Garden* says: "Masticate a little pepper or cardamom grains of the large species; put a certain quantity of it upon the head of your member and then go to work. This will produce for you, as well as for the woman, a matchless enjoyment."

Arabs add cardamom to beverages and drink the mixture as an aphrodisiac. They also sprinkle powdered cardamom, ginger, and cinnamon over boiled onions and green peas to promote erotic vigor. In India, powdered cardamom boiled with milk is consumed with honey at night to prevent impotence and premature ejaculation.

Cardamom in the Medicine Cabinet

Here are some common cardamom folk remedies.

- *Need a lift?* Cardamom contains a central nervous system stimulant called cineole and is used in traditional Chinese medicine to increase Qi (overall life force), improve mood, and generate strength.
- *Bad breath?* Combine cardamom (a potent antiseptic) with parsley, mint, and a cup of vodka and use as a mouthwash.
- *Got a rumbly tummbly?* Cardamom may help stop gas, heartburn, indigestion, and nausea. If you suffer from emphysema, try adding a teaspoon or two of powdered cardamom to fruit juice or tea—it's a potent expectorant.
- *Vaginal infection?* Cardamom contains a substance called terpinen-4-ol that fights yeast infections.
- *Have trouble digesting wheat?* Sprinkle cardamom on your cereal and bread and see if it helps.

Native to southern India and Sri Lanka, Egyptians chewed the pungent seeds to clean their teeth, and the ancient Romans, who prized the spice above all others, used cardamom as a perfume. Along with promoting love and sex cardamom is used to aid digestion, freshen the breath, and treat candida, emphysema, and obesity.

The warm, pungent, aromatic spice has a sweet, ginger-like flavor with eucalyptus and citrus overtones that make it perfect for savory dishes and baked goods. Ground cardamom seeds play a key role in Indian cuisine, where they are used to flavor everything from curries and rice pudding to chai and the yogurt drink lassi. Scandinavians incorporate cardamom into pastries and cakes and the Dutch use it in windmill biscuits.

When buying cardamom look for whole pods (which can be split and added to Indian dal or rice dishes or dropped whole in coffee or tea) or whole seeds, which can be ground and toasted alone or with other spices and used to flavor pilafs, vegetables, or meat dishes.

other sexy spices

clove

The dried flower buds of an evergreen tree in the myrtle family, clove has been used as an aphrodisiac in China since 300 B.C., when subjects chewed on cloves to sweeten their breath before meeting with the emperor. Cloves, because they are shaped like a tiny penis, are considered a sexual stimulant for men. The seventeenth-century Swedish herbalist Anders Mansson recommended that impotent men drink milk spiked with cloves.

The word *clove* comes from the Latin word for tack, *clovus*. Cloves have a warm, sweet, almost peppery flavor that is frequently used to add character to cakes, fruit compotes, mulled wine, and ham. Try adding ground cloves to gingerbread, cookies, apple sauce, muffins, maple syrup, and barbecue sauces. Whole cloves can be added to split pea and bean soups or poked into ham before cooking.

Ginger

Ginger, the fibrous root of *Zingiber officinale*, is used in Indian, Turkish, Arabian, and Oriental aphrodisiac potions internally and externally, often combined with honey and pepper. To combat impotence, Indian love manuals recommend eating ginger juice

spice Advice

To keep your spices tasting right you need to treat them with care. Under ideal conditions whole spices will stay fresh for up to two years; ground spices will keep for about six months. Here are some tips.

- Your neighborhood grocery store is great for milk and eggs, but it's not the place to purchase exotic spices. Buy spices from a store that specializes in them (natural food stores and ethnic markets are usually good bets) and has a quick turnover. Ask how often the store receives shipments of spices, and use your nose to smell how fresh the spices are.
- With the exception of cinnamon, which is hard to grind, buy whole spices and grind them yourself in a clean coffee bean grinder or with a mortar and pestle. Whole spices stay fresher longer, and freshly ground spices are more flavorful than previously ground spices.
- To intensify the flavor of your spices, roast them lightly in a dry skillet over medium-low heat for about 5 minutes, stirring occasionally.
- Store spices in a cool, dry place away from direct sunlight.

mixed with honey and half-boiled eggs. *The Perfumed Garden* has a recipe for a stimulating rub designed to drive women crazy. Just chew a mixture of ginger, cinnamon, cubeb, and pepper, and apply the compound to the penis before sex.

The Chinese believe ginger fruit jam works as an aphrodisiac. The fresh root, whose name comes from *sinabera,* a Sanskrit word that means "shaped like a horn," resembles an antler, and has long been considered an aphrodisiac because of its phallic shape.

During the nineteenth century, English pubs kept shakers of powdered ginger at the bar to sprinkle in beer, which eventually gave rise to the popular soft drink ginger ale. In Europe, young maidens baked and ate gingerbread men, believing the ritual would bring them a husband.

Crystallized ginger, which is made from sugared, dried ginger, can be eaten on its own or chopped and added to fruit salads, ice cream, smoothies, and baked goods.

Fresh gingerroot (look for it in the produce section near Asian groceries) can be grated, sliced, or chopped, and added to sauces, stir-fries, soups, and meat dishes such as roast chicken and pork tenderloin. The grated pulp can be squeezed in dishes as you would lemon juice, to brighten and sharpen flavors and add a little heat and fragrance. Chewing on crystallized ginger or sipping ginger tea made by pouring boiling water over sliced ginger is a great way to treat nausea (a British study found powdered ginger was twice as effective as Dramamine in preventing motion sickness), settle an upset stomach, or entice a lover.

nutmeg

The ripe, dried seed of *Myristica fragrans,* an evergreen tree native to the Molucca Islands in Southern Asia, which also produces mace, was highly valued in the Orient as well as among the Greeks, Romans, Arabs, and Hindus as an aphrodisiac. According to H. K. Bakhru, author of *Herbs that Heal,* nutmeg, when mixed with honey and a half-boiled egg, makes an excellent sex tonic that prolongs the duration of the sexual act if taken an hour before intercourse.

Nutmeg, eaten in large amounts, also has a slight hallucinogenic effect (nutmeg contains a compound called myristicin, which is similar to mescaline); however, the amounts required to make you high also will make you very sick. Our advice, stick to martinis.

Nutmeg trees have a gender. One male is needed for about every dozen female trees to ensure fertile fruit. The trees begin bearing fruit at around age ten and continue to be productive until they are between thirty and forty years old.

The sweet, pungent spice, which should be freshly grated right before use because the flavor disappears quickly after grating, is most frequently used as the finishing touch on egg nog. Nutmeg, a popular spice in Italy, Britain, and the Netherlands, is also used to flavor baked goods, sausages, soups, puddings, meats, stews, mashed potatoes, spinach, and fruit pies.

saffron

Reputedly saffron acts like a sex hormone and makes erogenous zones more sensitive. The Phoenicians offered moon-shaped, saffron-flavored love cakes to their fertility goddess Astoreth. According to Greek legend, eating saffron for a week would make a girl unable to resist a lover. One Arabic sex recipe calls for boiling saffron mixed with dates, anise, wild carrots, orange blossoms, and egg yolks in water mixed with honey and the blood of two freshly killed doves (Yum!). Saffron has also been used as a dye and as a perfume for Greek and Roman baths.

At around $50 per ounce, saffron is the world's most expensive spice. A Mediterranean native, it is made from the stigma of a flowering crocus called *Crocus sativus*. It takes about 4,000 to 5,000 hand-picked blossoms (more than 225,000 stigmas) to make one pound of the orange threads that are used to flavor French bouillabaisse, Scandinavian sweetbreads, Spanish paella, and Italian risotto. Fortunately, you only need a pinch of the intense, slightly bitter spice to flavor and color dishes and mellow your kitchen with saffron's strong fragrance.

From the moment primitive man noticed that certain parts of plants made meat taste better (approximately 50,000 years ago) to the present, people have enjoyed and craved herbs and spices as appetite and sexual stimulants. Today most spices are relatively inexpensive, and it's hard to believe that these pungent and powerful leaves, roots, and seeds were once so precious and difficult to find and import that men risked their lives and traveled the globe for a few pounds of pepper, cinnamon, or nutmeg. The allure of herbs and spices was so powerful that they formed the backbone of all great cuisines and still rule in the kitchen and the bedroom today.

Although supported more by mythology and folklore than science (with a few notable exceptions, such as parsley and the smell of cinnamon, especially when combined with ginger and clove), many cultures continue to believe that certain herbs and spices are endowed with aphrodisiacal powers.

The answer? You decide. Open your senses and taste, smell (remember, some smells are sexual turn-ons), experiment, and experience what herbs and spices have to offer and see what works for you. With a little practice you'll soon discover that accenting your life with these fragrant treasures can open up a whole new realm of exotic delights and erotic nights.

The cooking couple's herb and spice menu for amour

{ Ginger salad dressing }

1 (1-inch) piece of fresh ginger, grated
3 tablespoons vegetable oil
1 tablespoon toasted sesame oil
2 tablespoons rice vinegar
1 tablespoon soy sauce
1 tablespoon sugar
Mix all ingredients together and serve over salad.

{ Sexy mussels }

No, you don't get these mussels at the gym. But they might just get you the hard-bodied partner you've been looking for! Serve with plenty of ice-cold Belgian beer and crusty French bread.

1 tablespoon olive oil
1 medium onion, finely chopped
3 garlic cloves, minced
1 teaspoon grated gingerroot
1 teaspoon curry powder
2 pounds mussels, cleaned and debearded
⅓ cup Belgian beer (such as Hoegaarden or Stella Artois)
Freshly ground black pepper
2 tablespoons chopped cilantro

1. Heat the olive oil over medium heat in a pot large enough to hold all of the mussels. Add the onion and sauté until onion is translucent, about 5 minutes.
2. Add the garlic, gingerroot, and curry powder and sauté for another minute.
3. Add the beer and mussels. Cover tightly, increase heat to high, and steam mussels until they open, 3 to 4 minutes.
4. Ladle mussels and broth into soup bowls and sprinkle with cilantro. Sop up extra broth with bread.

{ Herb Roasted Potatoes }

1 pound new potatoes, cleaned and cut into quarters
2 tablespoons olive oil
1/2 teaspoon salt
1/4 teaspoon black pepper
2 tablespoons chopped fresh herbs
1. Preheat oven to 375° F.
2. Toss potatoes with olive oil, salt, and pepper. Roast in preheated oven until soft, about 30 minutes. Toss with fresh herbs and
   serve.

{ Spiced Honey Hens }

These tasty birds get their aphrodisiacal allure from garlic, ginger,
and five-spice powder, which is a blend of anise, clove, fennel, cinnamon, and Szechuan peppercorns.

2 Cornish game hens
3/4 cup honey
1 cup orange juice
1/4 cup soy sauce
2 garlic cloves, minced
1 tablespoon grated gingerroot
1/2 teaspoon five-spice powder

1. Wash hens well, both inside and out, and dry with paper towels.
   Butterfly the hens: Remove the backbone with kitchen shears or
   heavy chef's knife, and flatten the birds, breast side up, with palm
   of hand. Place in nonreactive bowl large enough to hold both
   hens.
2. In a small bowl, combine honey, orange juice, soy sauce, garlic,
   gingerroot, and five-spice powder. Pour over hens and cover. Let
   hens marinate for at least 2 hours or better yet, overnight, in the
   refrigerator. Turn occasionally to ensure even marination.
3. Remove hens from marinade. Boil marinade for at least 5 minutes
   to use for basting birds.

To grill: Preheat grill to medium. Set hens, skin side down, on an oiled grill grate and cook, basting occasionally, for 15 minutes or until skin is golden brown but not burned. Turn and grill until thoroughly cooked, about 15 minutes longer, basting occasionally.

To roast: Place oven rack in lower-middle position, and preheat oven to 400° F. Put the hens, skin side up, on a rack on top of a roasting or jelly roll pan. Roast hens, basting occasionally, until browned, about 25 minutes. Place birds under the broiler for a few minutes to crisp skin.

Serves 2

{ jerk chicken wings }

Turn up the reggae and pop a Red Stripe, 'cause we're gonna have some hot fun tonight.

1 medium onion, cut in quarters

1 bunch scallions

4 garlic cloves

1 (1-inch piece) gingerroot

1 to 4 jalapeño peppers (depending on how hot you want your wings)

Juice of one lime

1½ teaspoons dried thyme

1 teaspoon salt

1 teaspoon black pepper

1½ teaspoons ground allspice

¼ teaspoon nutmeg

½ teaspoon cinnamon

2 tablespoons soy sauce

¼ cup vegetable oil

16 chicken wings

1. In a food processor or blender, purée all ingredients except wings.
2. Place wings in a large nonreactive bowl or Ziploc bag and toss with jerk marinade. Cover and let wings marinate in the refrigerator for several hours or overnight.

3. Preheat oven to 425° F. Place wings in a pan, skin side up, and bake in top half of oven until cooked through, 30 to 35 minutes.

Serves 2 as a main course, 4 as an appetizer

{ Steak au Poivre }

For this classic French dish press the steaks into crushed black peppercorns and sprinkle the pan with a teaspoon of coarse salt before cooking.

2 tablespoons black peppercorns

1 teaspoon olive oil

2 filet mignon steaks, each ½ pound

Salt to taste

¼ cup red wine

1. Using a mortar and pestle, crush the peppercorns to a medium coarseness. Using the heel of your hand, press the crushed peppercorns into both sides of the steaks.
2. Heat a heavy frying pan over high heat and add olive oil.
3. Quickly sear the steaks on both sides. Reduce the heat to medium-high and cook about 3 minutes per side for medium rare.
4. Remove steaks to a warm platter. Season with salt. Cover and let rest for 5 minutes before serving.
5. While steaks are resting, pour wine into pan to deglaze. Cook for another minute and pour over steaks.

Serves 2

{ Fettuccine in a creamy Herb sauce }

This dish is so delicious that it's hard to believe it's actually low-cal.

4 ounces ham or prosciutto, thinly sliced

1 pound fettuccine

2 tablespoons olive oil

¼ cup chopped onion

1 (12-ounce) can evaporated skimmed milk

1 teaspoon lemon zest

¼ cup fresh basil leaves, chopped

¼ cup fresh parsley, chopped

1 tablespoon fresh mint leaves, chopped

¾ cup freshly grated Parmesan or Romano cheese

Salt and freshly ground black pepper to taste

1. Cut ham or proscuitto into thin (¼-inch wide), 2-inch-long strips and set aside.
2. Cook pasta in boiling salted water until al dente (literally "firm to the teeth").
3. While pasta is cooking, heat olive oil in a large sauté pan over medium heat. Sauté onion until soft, about 5 minutes.
4. Add evaporated skimmed milk and lemon zest to sauté pan and cook until milk is hot, 1 to 2 minutes. Remove pan from heat.
5. When pasta is done, drain, and add to sauté pan. Stir in the basil, parsley, mint, sliced ham or prosciutto, and cheese. Season with salt and freshly ground black pepper to taste and serve.

Serves 4

{ Double your Pleasure Gingerbread }

This intense bread gets its lively, stimulating flavor from a variety of aphrodisiacal spices, along with both crystallized and fresh ginger.

1⅔ cups all-purpose flour

½ teaspoon ground cinnamon

½ teaspoon ground cloves

½ teaspoon nutmeg

½ teaspoon cardamom

1 teaspoon baking soda

½ teaspoon salt

½ cup packed dark brown sugar

½ cup sugar

½ cup (1 stick) butter, room temperature

2 large eggs

2 tablespoons peeled, minced fresh gingerroot

¼ cup minced crystallized ginger

½ cup buttermilk

1. Preheat oven to 350° F.

2. Grease and flour an 8½ x 4½-inch loaf pan.

3. Sift together the first 7 ingredients and set aside.

4. Beat together the butter and sugars until light and fluffy. Beat in the eggs one at a time, followed by the crystallized ginger and fresh gingerroot.

5. Stir half of flour mixture into the butter/sugar/egg/ginger mixture. Stir in ¼ cup buttermilk, followed by the rest of the flour mixture, followed by the rest of the buttermilk.

6. Pour batter into prepared pan. Bake until bread springs back quickly when touched with a fork, about 50 minutes.

{ chocolate, coffee, and cardamom cheesecake }

An aphrodisiac triple-header so good, even dietitians indulge.

6 ounces chocolate chip cookies, finely crushed

¼ cup unsalted butter, melted

1 pound cream cheese

1¼ cups light cream

3 eggs

¼ cup flour

⅓ cup sugar

2 tablespoons strong black coffee

½ teaspoon ground cardamom

2 ounces dark chocolate

1. Preheat oven to 350° F.

2. Stir together crushed chocolate chip cookies and melted butter. Press into the bottom of a greased, 8-inch, springform pan.

3. Using an electric mixer, make filling by beating cream cheese with light cream until smooth. Add eggs, flour, sugar, coffee, and cardamom and beat together with mixer until thoroughly combined. Pour filling over crust.

4. Melt chocolate in microwave and drizzle over filling. For a marbled effect, swirl chocolate with the handle of a spoon.

5. Bake in preheated oven until firm, 50 to 60 minutes. Open oven door and allow cheesecake to cool. Release from pan, and chill in refrigerator for at least 2 hours before serving.

{ Camel's Milk Express }

"Camel's milk mixed with honey and taken regularly develops a vigor for copulation which is unaccountable and causes the virile member to be on the alert night and day," so says Sheikh Nefzaoui. Here's our version of his lusty beverage. If you can't find a camel to milk, substitute cow's or goat's milk. When ordering, specify one hump or two. Happy humping!

2 cups milk (camel, goat, or cow)

Pinch of saffron

Pinch of ground cardamom

Honey to taste

Gently warm milk in a saucepan. Add saffron, cardamom, and honey to taste. Pour into mugs and enjoy.

{ Turkish Coffee }

Brew up a buzz for your harem. Turkish coffee is traditionally made in a long-handled brass or copper pot called an ibrik. If you don't have one, a saucepan will do.

1½ cups water
4 heaping teaspoons espresso grind coffee
4 teaspoons sugar
Pinch of ground cardamom

1. Pour water in a small saucepan and bring to a boil over low heat.
2. Add coffee, sugar, and cardamom. Allow coffee to return to a slow boil. When mixture is thick and foamy, remove pan from heat and stir. Repeat the boiling, foaming, stirring step two more times and serve in demitasse (espresso) cups.

Serves 2

Herb and Spice Aphro-snacks

{ Herb Dip }

For a skinny dip, use reduced-fat cream cheese and low-fat sour cream or yogurt.

8 ounces cream cheese
¼ cup yogurt, sour cream, or crème fraîche
¼ cup chopped mixed herbs (such as parsley, basil, and thyme)
Salt and pepper to taste

Thoroughly combine all ingredients in a small bowl. Serve with cut-up vegetables.

{ curried ALmonds }

The combination of almonds and curry powder (a spice blend that contains many aphrodisiacs, including coriander, fennel, black pepper, ginger, cinnamon, garlic, mustard, and chiles) makes a glowing, crunchy, libido-boosting snack, perfect for refueling.

3 tablespoons butter

1 teaspoon curry powder

1½ cups whole almonds

1 teaspoon coarse salt

Preheat oven to 350° F. Melt butter over medium-low heat in a heavy saucepan. Add curry powder and cook, stirring occasionally, for 2 to 3 minutes. Add almonds and stir to coat. Spread almonds on a rimmed baking sheet and toast in preheated oven for 15 minutes. Toss with salt, cool, and enjoy.

9
Edible orgy

Now it's time to put your newfound expertise to work. This book is about fun, so start having some. It's time to plan your own edible orgy!

Don't get nervous, we'll hold your hand. Besides, it's pretty easy. Just follow our step-by-step instructions and get ready for romance, love, and lust. (And great food, too!)

orgy worship

While today we think of orgies as wild sex parties, orgies were originally ceremonial rites that were held in honor of ancient Greek and Roman deities. In fact, modern theater actually originated in Athens, and came from the ceremonial orgies of Dionysus, the Greek god of wine and fertility.

In ancient times sexuality and eroticism were accepted and celebrated as a basic human and universal life force. There was no shame in being sexually active. Prostitutes were invited to parties, and ecstatic singing, dancing, and lovemaking were forms of worship. At feasts, festivals, banquets, and weddings, servants, cup bearers, dancers, and other entertainers frequently served and performed naked or dressed in provocative clothing to help excite sexual desire and honor the gods.

Famous orgies included:

·Aphrodisia, a popular Greek festival honoring Aphrodite, the goddess of love. As part of the celebration, women aroused men with lewd attire, talk, and gestures, while prostitutes and their companions, who were called hetaerae, honored the goddess by having sex.

- Saturnalia, the winter solstice festival honoring Saturn, the Roman god of agriculture. The harvest was in, nights were long, it was between seasons, people were bored, and they decided it was time to party. As Roman culture became more unrestrained and licentious, so did Saturnalia. Here's how Seneca the Younger describes Rome during one first-century Saturnalia.

> . . . take a better supper and throw off the toga.

- Alexander VI was one pope who knew how to pop the cork. One of the richest men of his day and possibly the most notorious pope ever, Alexander threw the most lavish orgies of the Renaissance. The wild Vatican parties—which included animals, whores, and church officials—were costly affairs. Here's how Voltaire describes some of the festivities.

> As guests approached the papal palace, they were excited by the spectacle of living statues: naked, gilded young men and women in erotic poses. Inside, candelabra were set up on the floor, scattered among them were chestnuts, which the courtesans had to pick up, crawling between the candles. Then the guests stripped and ran out onto the floor, where they mounted, or were mounted by, the prostitutes. Servants kept score of each man's orgasms, for the pope greatly admired virility, and measured a man's machismo by his ejaculative capacity. After everyone was exhausted, his Holiness distributed prizes—cloaks, boots, caps, and fine silken tunics. The winners were those who made love with the courtesans the greatest number of times.

pLanning your EdibLe orgy

This is a time to indulge and enjoy yourself and the one you love or lust after. So make sure you have the time and space for fun.

This is not a lunchtime quickie. It is a long, lounging, self-indulgent, decadent day of culinary delights and sensual heights that is your reward for all the hard work, stress, and pressure you endure.

If you've got kids, call the in-laws and cash in all the baby-sitting chits. No in-laws? First, lucky you. Next, see if a friend can take the kids overnight or at least for a long afternoon. If all else fails, do what we do. Rent the two longest Disney films you can find (we use *Fantasia* and all the Dalmatians films, *101, 102,* both live and animated versions). Set the kids up in front of the TV with their favorite snacks. Tell them if they need Mommy or Daddy to come to the bottom of the stairs and yell, and then keep your fingers crossed and start serving, and cooking, in the bedroom. In our research we have found that Disney is 75 percent effective for up to three hours. A tip: Don't start the films until all food is prepared and ready to go. You don't want to blow a half hour of privacy opening oysters and shaking martinis.

Ah, yes, we hear the politically correct screams from the back of the room. "Put the kids in front of TV? That's horrible." "You're rotting their brains." "Disney reinforces stereotypes." "You're being selfish." "You should use the time for teaching them," etc. Well, guess what: Parenting is the most underpaid, overworked, unappreciated, psychologically challenging, and personally satisfying job there is. And everyone, even parents, deserves a break once in a while. Happy parents are better parents, and the best way we know to stay happy and in love is to take the time to treat each other to some fun, satisfaction, and heightened endorphin levels. There is nothing wrong with showing your partner you love them and there is nothing wrong with enjoying great sex. According to a study done by Plechaty, Couturier, Cote, Roy et al., intimacy and communication (which play a very important role in great sex) are major influences on a couple's marital satisfaction.

Believe us, our kids think we're a lot more fun when we emerge from our lair with happy grins slapped across our faces than when Daddy comes stalking downstairs muttering, "You talkin' to me?"

If they're old enough, give the kids movie money, drop them off at the multiplex or mall, and pick them up later. If they're teenagers, you're in luck. The last place they want to be is home with you, so it should be no problem getting rid of them for long periods of time. The problem is getting them to come back when you're done.

If you're single, living together, or married without kids, ignore the preceding and . . . let the games begin.

Theme of your EdibLe orgy

Michael prefers the elegant orgy scenario. Ellen, being the Francophile in the family, prefers the lavish and overindulgent eighteenth-century French style of decadence. Later in this chapter, we give you themed edible orgies for all tastes.

Don't let our list stop you. If we don't mention one you like, then design your own. Maybe you like the Geisha-Samurai Sushi Party, or the President/Intern scenario. Whatever you choose, it's all about fun, so let your imagination and libido run wild.

PLanning the Menu for your EdibLe orgy

You don't have to. We've done all the work for you already. All you have to do is shop. However, if you're one of those anti-authoritarian types who has to make all of the decisions themselves, go ahead, plan your own menu. Just keep these tips in mind.

1. All recipes should be quick, simple, and as foolproof as possible.

2. Optimize flexibility. This means creating dishes that can sit in the fridge for an hour or two before being served or quickly heated. Don't design your menu around dishes, like soufflé, that must be eaten right away. Focus on dishes you can make

ahead of time. Trust us. This is not about chopping, slicing, and dicing. We want to get you out of the kitchen and into the bedroom.

3. Eat foods that you and your lover like. Sounds simple, but you'd be surprised how many people serve foods that they dislike just to impress. It's your party, so have fun. If chocolate-covered gummy bears turn you on and caviar doesn't, skip the roe and go dipping.

4. Be creative. Design a menu that ignites all the senses and offers plenty of variety and contrasts in terms of color, texture, temperature, and flavor.

5. Lite is right. Don't weigh yourself and your lover down with heavy, hard-to-digest foods that will take energy away from lovemaking. Entice your lover with beautiful food and seductive tastes, textures, and aromas, not fat and calories.

6. Think finger foods. Eating with your hands is inherently sexy. After all, someone has to lick those fingers clean!

7. To maximize your love buzz, make sure to include plenty of aphrodisiacs on your menu.

shopping for your edible orgy

Try not to wait until the day of your edible orgy to shop. Have everything done the day before so you can concentrate on preparing, relaxing, and getting and staying in the mood. The only shopping that should be left to orgy day is for food that must be prepared and served fresh, such as shellfish or sushi.

serving your edible orgy

For our edible orgies we prefer to stick with foods that fit into the "grazing tray" category. These are foods you can prep, place on platters and plates, and nibble on throughout the day, evening, night, or if you're really lucky, the weekend. We don't recommend that you drag yourself out of bed or off the floor to cook and eat a roast duck with an oriental aphrodisiacal spice rub. If you really want duck (which goes great with champagne or a good Pinot Noir), cook it earlier and serve it cool. (Yes, duck tastes great cool.) The food should not rule you; you rule the food. That's why nuts, fresh fruit, cheese, chocolate, oysters, shrimp, and caviar are such great edible orgy foods. You want to be able to refuel quickly with high-energy, great-tasting, sensual foods that contain aphrodisiacs.

Enjoying Your EdibLe orgy

We recommend nibbling over a long period of time, punctuated with bouts of energetic sex and orgasmically induced endorphin highs. Then, use your edible orgy to satiate your hunger, refuel your lust tank, and keep the endorphins up for more fun.

RefueLing

There are stimulants that provide both quick and sustained energy for sexual refueling, increase endorphin levels, arouse the libido, and get into your bloodstream quickly, providing your sexual machinery with the chemicals needed to rejuvenate rapidly for another fun run. Here are a few of our favorites:
·Chocolate
·Shellfish (particularly oysters)
·Caviar
·Black licorice or a licorice-flavored drink
·Fruit, particularly fresh figs, grapes, mangoes, bananas, and strawberries
·Small amounts of beef
·Pumpkin seeds
·Coffee

If you want to know how and why these sexually stimulating foods work, just check out the chapter where each is mentioned in this book.

There's Got to Be a Morning After . . .

Chinese food makes great morning-after snacks, and so do aphrodisiacs. How about some cinnamon buns, a sexual smoothie (try our recipes for Estrogen Elixir, Testosterone Tornado, or Creamy Coffee Avocado Shake), or Arabic Egg Mash with that morning cup of coffee? (Studies have shown that coffee drinkers are more sexually active than non-coffee drinkers.) Just because the sun's up doesn't mean the party has to stop. There's nothing wrong with a morning sex snack. It might just turn into a sexual brunch.

The Cooking Couple's Favorite Edible Orgy Scenarios

Here are some of our favorite edible orgy menus. Feel free to mix and match your favorites, or design your own using the foods we talk about in the book. An edible orgy is all part of foreplay. That's *for play*! So play. Feed your libido correctly, and it will treat you to great enjoyment, fulfillment, and lots of endorphin highs for years to come.

Caribbean Blue Holiday Orgy

You put the lime in the coconut and drink it all up.

Aphrodisiacs are sold throughout the Caribbean at roadside stands and markets. If you want to be really authentic, start with mannish water (also called power water), a spicy soup made from goat's head, garlic, scallions, green bananas, and Scotch bonnet peppers. (For an extra kick, white rum or Irish Moss, an island aphrodisiac for men made from seaweed extract, is sometimes added.) You might also order Bois Bandé (French for "hard wood"), the bark of a tree that grows in the Caribbean, famous for enhancing male performance. You can make a tea from the bark or place a piece of bark in a bottle of rum and let the mixture stand for a few weeks before drinking.

For those of you who can't get to the Caribbean and don't have access to goat heads, Irish Moss, or Bois Bandé, bring the Caribbean home. Turn up the heat to 80 degrees, play your favorite reggae CD, and put on that special bikini or Hawaiian shirt. Here's a hot Caribbean holiday orgy menu that will take your endorphin levels higher and higher.

caribbean bLue HoLiday orgy menu

*Ginger beer, Corona with lime, Rum Runners,
or your favorite summer cocktail (Banana Daiquiri,
Sex on the Beach, etc.)
Caribbean Crostini (recipe page 134)
Hot, Hot, Hot Shrimp Cocktail
Jerk Chicken Wings (recipe page 251)
Aphro Fruit Salsa with chips (recipe page 184)
Hot Mango Ice Cream (recipe page 139)*

game pLan

1 to 24 hours ahead of time

•Make the Hot Mango Ice Cream.
•Make the Jerk Chicken Wings.
•Prepare the crostini topping and cut French bread.
•Defrost one pound cooked cocktail shrimp in the refrigerator.
•Spike the cocktail sauce with a dash of Caribbean hot sauce to taste.
•Make the Aphro Fruit Salsa.
•Chill chosen beverages or mixers.

Party Time

·Take out shrimp and cocktail sauce. Place shrimp on nice platter.
·Finish crostini and place on platter.
·Take out chicken wings. Serve cold, or reheat quickly in microwave.
·Serve Aphro Fruit Salsa with chips.
·Serve beverages. For the Rum Runners, mix 1 cup pineapple juice with 1 cup orange juice, 1 cup ginger ale, and ½ cup dark rum. Add 1 tablespoon grenadine and 1 tablespoon lime juice.
·Don't forget to eat the Mango Ice Cream as a mid-orgy refresher.

Want to really send those endorphins through the roof? Get out the hot sauce and see which of you is better able to take the heat. Or spread out the beach blanket, give each other hot coconut oil massages, and progress to even hotter lovemaking. Then cool off with a romantic Caribbean-inspired movie, such as Lina Wertmuller's *Swept Away* starring Giancarlo Giannini and Mariangela Melato as shipwrecked opposites forced into an uneasy alliance to satisfy their mutual lust.

The Elegant Edible Orgy

The Rat Pack is back and 1950s-style elegance is in the air tonight. You play Heff. She plays the Bunny. And you both get to peel the carrot as Frank, Dino, and Sammy croon finger-poppin' tunes to the beat of a martini shaker. This is a classy black tie affair, but that doesn't mean he has to wear pants. (Maybe that's why it's Michael's favorite.) Remember, boys, bunnies love to be scratched behind their ears.

The Elegant Edible Orgy Menu

Champagne or bone-dry vodka martinis
Caviar and oysters

Mixed greens
Asparagus-Stuffed Steak
(About six ounces each. You don't want to
be too stuffed to . . .) (recipe page 219)
Cabernet Sauvignon wine
French bread
Cheese platter featuring Stilton and cheddar
Port
Assorted chocolates
Sorbet
Back to bed

Game PLan

1 to 24 hours ahead of time

·For this scenario we recommend a naked, postcoital, candlelit, sit-down dinner. Set the table ahead of time and pull out your favorite CDs. We recommend Sinatra, Tony Bennett, Diana Krall, Joe Henderson, Dinah Washington, Ella Fitzgerald (especially when she sings Cole Porter), and Charlie Haden.
·Prep steak so it is ready for roasting.
·Make salad.

30 minutes ahead of time

·Open the oysters and let them sit on ice in the refrigerator.
·Let the steak come to room temperature and preheat oven.
·Place cheeses on a plate and let them come to room temperature.
·Dress (or undress) for dinner.

Party time

- Put steak in preheated oven.
- Turn on the tunes. Open the champagne. Feed each other oysters and caviar.
- Open the wine. Place salads, wine, and bread on table. Nibble on your salads and bread and have a glass of wine while steak cooks.
- Take steak out of oven. Let steak rest for 10 minutes. Slice steak and serve.
- Serve cheese course with port.
- Serve dessert and coffee.

So you wanna be a rock and roll star? Edible orgy

What's your name, little girl, what's your name?
Couldn't you stay, little girl, and have a drink of champagne?

—Lynyrd Skynyrd

Did you always want to be Mick Jagger? Did you always want to say "I'm with the band"? Here's an all-night rock and roll party for two. Better clear your calendar for tomorrow because if you're gonna live the life, then this party goes to sunup, and the two of you get to lounge around in a dreamy haze snacking on aphrodisiacs, each other, and champagne all day long until the limo arrives for the next gig. And don't forget to bring the attitude, mate: "Only a magnum of champagne? You must be daft, you bloody bugger! Never mind the bollocks, where's the absinthe?"

so you wanna Be a Rock and RoLL star? orgy Menu

Champagne
Lobster
Black licorice and jelly bean shooters

These cocktails are designed to keep him up all night long (recipes page 156).

Licorice whips
Mini bar munch out
Leather and Silk Ice Cream (recipe page 159)
Cold pizza with assorted aphrodisiac toppings

Game PLan

1 to 24 Hours Ahead of Time

• Prepare lobster: Boil him up ahead of time or have your fish market cook it for you so all you have to do is melt the butter, dip, and slurp. Cold lobster tastes great.

• Make the Leather and Silk ice cream.

• Chill the champagne: Just to be showy, true rock and rollers would order the most expensive champagne on the room service menu. We recommend you splurge on some Möet White Star (not too expensive, but it tastes like it is).

• Stock the mini bar. Any real groupie will tell you 4 A.M. is the time to munch out at the in-room mini bar. So stock your home mini bar now with plenty of aphrodisiacal nibbles to keep your party going till sunup. Here's a list of some of our favorites:

  • M&M's

  • Good & Plenty, cucumbers, and banana nut bread, all of which increase vaginal blood flow in women.

  • Fresh fruit, especially bananas (very suggestive) and citrus fruit (refreshing after sex).

•Nuts and seeds, especially pine nuts (used in ancient and Medieval times as an aphrodisiac) and pumpkin seeds (rich in sexually stimulating nutrients).

•Wine

•Cheese and crackers (nine out of ten groupies prefer processed spreads, small individually wrapped cheeses, and Triskets).

•Hot Nuts (recipe page 137), Curried Almonds (recipe page 257), or Lite Chile Mix (recipe page 138) to keep the night smoking.

Party time

•Melt butter and set out with lobsters and nutcrackers.

•Open champagne and enjoy with lobster.

•Make licorice drinks and raid mini bar.

•For entertainment, tie each other up with licorice whips and eat your way to freedom.

•Feed each other Leather and Silk ice cream in bed.

The Morning After

The rock and roll breakfast of champions? Cold pizza, with aphrodisiacal toppings. Choose from: garlic, hot peppers, onions (raw or cooked), tomatoes, cooked asparagus, and/or canned artichoke hearts. Buy it the night before and eat cold in the A.M. Or drag yourselves to the corner joint for a romantic (and aphrodisiacal) eye opener of coffee and a pie. Then it's back to the sack for another snack!

Arabian Nights EdibLe orgy

*Midnight at the oasis
Send your camel to bed*

—Lyrics by David Nichtern,
sung by Maria Muldaur

For an Arabian night of erotic delights that last forever, get out the veil, turban, belly dancing music, and Turkish coffee, because it's time to rub the magic lamp and see what wishes that genie is granting tonight.

To set the stage for your desert romance: Lower the lights, drape a scarf over a lamp, and perfume your bedroom and your bodies with fragrant essential oils (if you are trying to be authentic, follow the recommendations of *The Perfumed Garden* and use a mixture of myrrh, rose, and musk). Have your sheikh park his camel on the bed next to you as you feed each other stuffed grape leaves, hummus, olives, dates, and pomegranate seeds. Use plenty of parsley, mint, and pepper in your yogurt dip, and a healthy dash of cardamom in your Turkish coffee.

Your bedroom will be hotter than the Sahara in July and your body will be his oasis.

Arabian Nights EdibLe orgy Menu

*Arabian Nights grazing tray: Hummus,
stuffed grape leaves, pita
bread, olives, dates, and pomegranates.
Camel's Milk Express (recipe page 255)
Baklava
Turkish Coffee (recipe page 256)*

The Game Plan

1 to 24 hours ahead of time

·Buy foods for your grazing tray. (Look for them in grocery stores that carry Middle Eastern specialty foods.)

Party time

·Put Arabian Nights grazing tray items on a platter.
·Make Camel's Milk Express.
·Feed each other items either in bed or on a carpeted floor.
·Serve postcoital Turkish Coffee and baklava.
·Try a little belly dancing and read each other *Tales from the Arabian Nights.* Then re-enact one of the tales. Extra slave girls and eunuchs are optional.

For the morning after, we recommend Arabic Egg Mash (Scrambled Eggs with Onion and Spices, recipe page 217) derived from a recipe recommended by Sheikh Nefzaoui, author of *The Perfumed Garden,* along with pita bread served with melted butter and honey, and more Turkish Coffee. Then, it's off to the aphrodisiac bazaar to refuel the camel for the next caravan. Take your fill of love until the morning sun is high in the sky, and rock the casbah till the moon shows bright in the desert night.

The Model and Her Boy Toy Edible Orgy

I'm too sexy for myself, too sexy for myself, and everyone else!

–Right Said Fred, "I'm Too Sexy"

Light and tight is the way a model likes it. Although it seems like these creatures of the catwalk survive on nothing more than cigarettes and celery sticks, when it comes to partying there's a reason that models are referred to as "girls behaving badly." Here's a high-fashion menu that keeps the calories low, libido-enhancing chemicals high, and sensuality front and center.

So strap on your Jimmy Choo mules, put on something short, skimpy, and see-through, and put your boy toy through his paces. If he's a good puppy, throw him a juicy steak and let him kiss your toes!

THE MODEL AND HER BOY TOY EDIBLE ORGY MENU

For those of you watching your calories, this one can also function as your diet/low-fat orgy menu.

Champagne
Raw oysters on the half shell with Tabasco sauce if you
like it hot, or caviar if you like it cool
Assorted crudités (cut-up vegetables)
with
Herb Dip (recipe page 256)
Strawberries with fat-free chocolate syrup for
dipping, licking, drawing, and sticking
More champagne

THE GAME PLAN

1 to 24 hours ahead of time

•Wash and cut up vegetables. Be sure to include some of these aphrodisiacs: celery, carrots (the Greeks called carrots *philtorn,* and believed they were a love medicine. They are also a good source of beautifying beta carotene), steamed asparagus, mushrooms (they were served at Roman wedding feasts), and fennel.
•Make dip.
•Refrigerate champagne.

30 to 60 minutes ahead of time

•Wash and dry strawberries and put in an attractive bowl. Fill a
small bowl with chocolate sauce for dipping.
•Place vegetables on a platter.

Party Time!

•Take vegetables, dip, oysters, strawberries, and chocolate sauce
out of the refrigerator.
•Open oysters. Place them on a bed of ice.
•Don't forget to open the champagne. Champagne has 10 percent
fewer calories than Chardonnay, so have another glass.

For the true model or model wannabe, this scenario is not only
low in calories, it actually helps you lose weight. Here's how:

*2 glasses of champagne (170 calories) + 6 oysters with Tabasco
or caviar (58 calories) + crudités and dip (150 calories) + strawberries (60 calories) + chocolate syrup (46 calories) = 486 calories*

Subtract one night of fabulous sex (3 to 4 bouts of vigorous
lovemaking in an evening can easily burn 400 calories), and your
net total is a mere 86 calories. Just enough to keep a supermodel's
heart beating. ("You mean these chicks actually have hearts?")

The Classic French Edible Orgy
(Also known as the Marquis de Sade Special)

This is Ellen's favorite. Grab your wig and all the frilly underwear
you can put your hands on, and don't forget the corset, 'cause in
this one you're going back to eighteenth-century France and all
the decadence and lust that the marquis and his "friends" enjoyed. Minus little inconveniences like the French Revolution,
the guillotine, the plague, and lack of refrigeration, of course.
Quote the marquis, "A plenteous meal produces voluptuous sensations."

The Classic French Edible orgy Menu

Pâté de foie gras truffé (Goose or duck liver paté
with truffles)
(you can buy these items on the Internet or
in some upscale gourmet markets) with
Sauternes or Gewürztraminer wine
or
Brie with
French Bordeaux or Burgundy wine
Steak au Poivre (recipe page 252)
or
Chicken with 40 Cloves of Garlic (recipe page 218)
with
Artichokes or asparagus
Either Red Burgundy or Bordeaux for the beef
Syrah or Côtes du Rhône for the Chicken
Herb Roasted Potatoes (recipe page 250)
Hot chocolate
Assorted French pastries

Game Plan

1 to 24 hours ahead of time

·Make chicken.
·Roast potatoes.
·Set table.

30 to 60 minutes ahead of time

·Take out pâté or Brie.
·Prepare asparagus or artichokes for steaming.
·Chill white wine.

Party time

·Open wine and enjoy pâté or Brie.
·Heat up potatoes in microwave.
·Heat up chicken in microwave.
·Steam asparagus or artichokes.
·Cook steak (this only takes about 5 minutes) while you continue enjoying pâté or Brie.
·Serve cooked steak or chicken with potatoes and asparagus or artichokes.
·Serve hot chocolate and pastries after main course.

This luscious menu overflows with foods famous for their ability to arouse. We've already told you about chocolate, asparagus, and wine. Here are a few other love foods you should know about.

Foie gras. Foie gras, literally "fat liver," was enjoyed as an aphrodisiac by the French and Greeks. While foie gras can come from geese or ducks, goose liver is a more potent love food because geese are considered phallic (due to their long necks) and are linked with Aphrodite.

Truffles. Dubbed "the diamonds of cookery" by Brillat-Savarin, truffles, whose power to arouse comes from their musky aroma, have longed been hailed as an aphrodisiac. The Romans dedicated the prized fungus (mushrooms are considered a fungus) to Venus, and the Greeks believed they were created by thunderbolts. According to an old proverb: "Those who wish to live virtuous lives should abstain from truffles."

Artichokes. In France, artichokes, which are the flower bud of a thistle, were believed to heat the body, spirit, and genitals. According to Greek myth, Zeus, king of the gods, turned Cynara, an attractive young woman who refused his advances, into an artichoke, hence, the Latin name for artichokes is *Cynara scolymus.*

Catherine de Médicis, queen of France, was considered scandalous by the French court for eating large quantities of artichokes. Her husband, Henry, didn't seem to mind.

Filet mignon (used to make steak au poivre). The French writer and physician François Rabelais referred to the female genitals as *Mignon D'Amourette,* and *mignonne* is French slang for a rubenesque whore.

The Geisha-Samurai Sushi Orgy

You wanna kimono tonight? Don't let your samurai forget his sword because it's going to get sharp with these oriental aphrodisiac delights.

This one is the easiest of the bunch. All the geisha or samurai host has to do is buy an array of delectable sushi dishes, some instant miso soup mix, and a bottle of saki (rice wine), make a simple salad, and introduce Ling Ling to Ding Ding.

For sushi, we recommend anago (conger eel), hamaguri (clam), awabi (abalone), ebi (boiled shrimp), ikura (salmon roe), sake (salmon), tako (octopus), uni (sea urchin roe), and negitoro-maki (scallion-and-tuna roll). Take a look at our seafood chapter for all the info you need as to why these Japanese delights ignite love at night. If you are really ambitious, try out our aphro roll recipe (page 44). And don't forget the wasabi (Japanese horseradish) and gari (vinegared ginger), both of which are aphrodisiacs. For dessert we recommend green tea and vanilla ice cream topped with chopped, crystallized ginger.

Geisha-Samurai Sushi Orgy Menu

Sake
Salad with Ginger Salad Dressing (See recipe, page 249)
Miso soup

Assorted sushi
Crystallized ginger ice cream
Green tea

1 to 12 hours ahead of time

•Purchase sushi the day of the orgy. Many upscale grocery stores and natural food stores sell sushi, as well as miso paste or miso soup mix. If you can't find it in a grocery store, order take out from a Japanese restaurant. We recommend buying approximately two dozen à la carte pieces plus two different rolls (maki). If sushi doesn't come with appropriate condiments (wasabi, pickled ginger, and soy sauce) purchase separately.
•Buy sake and a sake set if you don't have one already. Chill sake.
•Make salads and dressing.

Party time

•Place sushi on platters and set on table.
•Pour dressing over salads and serve.
•Make soup, following package directions, and serve.
•Pour each other sake. (It is bad luck to pour your own.)

Passion can hit quickly, so put on your favorite kimonos (or bathrobes) and enjoy dinner seated on the floor around a low coffee table. To keep the sexual energy flowing, try Shiatsu, a Japanese massage technique that uses finger pressure to get energy, called chi, flowing. What flows after that is up to you.

The President and the Intern Edible Orgy

Serve cold pizza with aphrodisiacal herbs and spices on the office desk to replenish the prowess of the presidential probius. Round out the scene with some thong underwear, a navy Gap dress, and a cigar, and the party goes on until the Senate is back in session. Fruit, particularly over-ripe peaches, are a nice touch for dessert. Hail to the chief!

10

The Cooking Couple's Best Sex Diet: Eating to Optimize Your Sexual Vitality

In Hollywood they say it all starts with the script. In sex it's the body. Take care of it and it will take care of you and your orgasms for life. An apple, an oyster, and a walnut a day can keep you hard and ready for play. As a side benefit, it may keep the cardiologist and urologist away as well.

If your body is maintained, fueled, and garaged properly, it will perform like a sexual Rolls-Royce. If you're living on cigarettes, cola, and fast food and not taking time to relax and refuel your engine (that includes your psychological engine), then you've got a sexual jalopy destined for the scrap heap.

No matter what shape you're in, the Cooking Couple's Best Sex Diet Plan will have you off to the races in just a week. It's a healthy eating regimen with supplements that will naturally optimize sexual passion, pleasure, and performance.

Most diets tell you to stop eating to get in shape. But if it's sexual shape—great sex—that you're seeking, you're in for a treat. Just change your diet by *adding* key aphrodisiacs and nutrients and limit your intake of libido-quashing grub. No weight lifting, gym memberships, or gravity-defying yoga pretzel positions required.

A study analyzing sex in over 6,000 marriages and published in *The Journal of Sex Research* concluded that sexually inactive marriages are not happy, satisfying unions. A ten-year survey of 3,500 people in the United States and Europe found that people who have sex regularly look and feel younger.

Better Health = Better Sex, Better Sex = Better Health

Better overall health adds up to better sex. And, in turn, great sex boosts health, energy, circulation, and emotional well-being.

Orgasms are good medicine.

Keeping sexually active keeps your sex hormones (the chemical messengers that tell your body how to respond sexually) flowing. When hormones are balanced and abundant, your body responds promptly to sexual stimuli and you have more pleasurable, powerful, and erotic experiences.

Besides, sex is great aerobic exercise. The average lovemaking session burns 100 calories. Have sex three times a week for a year, and you'll burn 15,600. That's four and a half pounds!

Know another weight-loss program that's this much fun?

Great sex is good for everybody. Here's how to get it.

The Four Key Elements to Sexual Success

For both men and women, great sex depends on four primary elements:

1. Good head (a brain that responds to sexual stimuli).
2. Good chemistry (the correct balance of hormones and neurotransmitters).
3. Good circulation (a well-functioning cardiovascular system).
4. Good nutrition (so the body has the physical ability and energy to perform at its sexual peak).

Frequent sex is Good medicine

Here's what sex three times a week can do for you:
1. Increase testosterone levels (which will boost your sexual desire) and estrogen levels.
2. Enhance circulation and increase blood flow to all parts of the body so organs, cells, and muscles are nourished and oxygenated.
3. Reduce your risk of heart disease. Like any form of regular exercise, sex can help improve your cholesterol level (raise good HDL cholesterol and may lower bad LDL cholesterol), help you maintain a healthy weight, improve the fitness of your heart, and help keep blood pressure low.
4. Maintain a healthy prostate.
5. Provide a natural high and pain relief through the release of the body's natural opiates, endorphins.
6. Decrease stress, increase relaxation, and improve sleep.
7. Slow the aging process and increase longevity.
8. Boost the immune system.
9. Improve self-esteem.

What are you waiting for?

Good Head

The brain is the body's most important sex organ. The old adage that some men "think with their dicks" is false. Without the hypothalamus, the area of the brain that governs hormone production, the penis is useless.

The brain rules both desire and emotion and is the key that turns on the sexual spigot. If your brain doesn't respond to sexual stimuli (whether visual, auditory, tactile, or olfactory), your sexual gears stay stuck in neutral.

In first gear, your brain picks up the sexual scent. Apocrine glands around the groin area and in the armpits produce human pheromones, chemicals that send out a scent and that signal sex is on the menu. The brain then sends "Prepare for *sex*!!!" signals to the rest of the body via neurotransmitters and hormones (such as testosterone, which triggers the sex drive in both men and women).

Your heart beats faster, adrenaline and vaginal secretions flow, genitals become engorged with blood, the brain releases endorphins, you get excited and start to feel . . . (forgive us for using overly technical terms) horny, randy, hot, juiced up. . . .

Good Circulation

In order for men to attain and maintain an erection and for women to feel increased warmth, sensitivity, and sexual arousal, the body has to be able to pump blood effectively, especially to the genitals. For that, the cardiovascular (circulatory) system must be in shape.

Blood is like oil that flows through your car's engine. If your arteries are clogged, blood flow is impeded and the entire body, especially sexual responsiveness, becomes sluggish. It gets harder and harder (or should we say softer and softer?) to have an erection, and sexual stamina diminishes until . . . it's time to blow "Taps" for Mr. Happy, who is by now a very sad and lonely fellow.

Luckily, this story need not have a sad ending. It's never too late to reverse the problem. You can improve blood flow throughout your body without drugs or surgery by following our plan.

When you add aphrodisiacs to a healthy diet, it's like adding jet fuel to that Rolls. C'mon, make Mr. Happy happy again.

Good Chemistry

You may have failed chemistry in school, but we're going to make sure you get an A+ in sexual Chem 101 right now.

Great sex is all about good chemistry. When two people are

mutually attracted, we say they have "good chemistry" because sexual arousal is transmitted from our brains to our bodies by chemical messengers called hormones (manufactured by the endocrine glands) and neurotransmitters (manufactured from amino acids and generated in nerve cells).

Many aphrodisiacs work because they help keep the nervous and endocrine systems healthy and provide the nutritional building blocks to make hormones and neurotransmitters.

The body's endocrine system makes three types of sex hormones, androgens (male), estrogens (female, responsible for vaginal lubrication), and progesterone (female). The word *hormone* actually comes from the Greek word *hormōn,* which means to "stir up."

In response to sexual stimuli, the brain signals endocrine glands to release hormones that initiate sexual arousal. While men produce about ten times more testosterone than women (though a woman's level often rises near the time of ovulation), testosterone triggers libido in both sexes.

Arousal causes the brain to send signals via neurotransmitters, such as dopamine and adrenaline, through our nervous system to prepare the body for sex. One set of neurotransmitters sends messages to relax blood vessels in the genitals so that penile and vaginal tissues can become engorged with blood and erect, another set increases tension and overall excitement (heart rate, blood pressure, and sweating all increase) and makes ejaculation possible.

The right balance of neurotransmitters is essential for great sex. Now, for your final exam. Go have sex.

Good Nutrition

Okay, your brain is alert and sending signals via neurotransmitters to your body to prepare for sex. Your endocrine glands are churning out all the necessary hormones to make sex possible. And your heart is pumping extra blood through clean arteries so

BaLancing Yin and Yang

To have an orgasm you need to be excited, responsive, and alert to get aroused, but at the same time you need to be relaxed so that your body can be receptive to sexual pleasure and orgasm.

Many aphrodisiacs work by optimizing the balance of excitement (triggered by the sympathetic nervous system) and relaxation (triggered by the parasympathetic nervous system).

Expansive foods and beverages such as wine, tofu, and fruit can help relax a lover who is tense and tight, while contractive foods such as coffee, meat, and eggs can help increase alertness and excitement.

To enhance sexual satisfaction, it is best to balance expansive and contractive foods and use them in small amounts. You can experiment by trying out two classic aphrodisiac combinations: oysters (a contractive food) and beer (an expansive beverage), or caviar (a contractive food) and champagne (an expansive beverage).

that your genitals can become engorged with blood and erect. Now all you need for great sex is high-octane fuel for energy and stamina.

Good nutrition is the cornerstone of any sexual fitness program. A healthy, balanced diet that's low in saturated fat, trans fat, and cholesterol, and high in fiber, complex carbohydrates, essential fats, high-quality protein, and fresh fruits and vegetables provides the body with quality fuel and the raw materials to build the hormones and neurotransmitters needed for mattress-shattering sex. Eating right also promotes good circulation and keeps your body at a healthy weight, making you more attractive and better able to perform sexually. According to a Duke University Diet and Fitness Center study, people who lost weight reported feeling increased sexual desire. A healthy diet can also help prevent obesity, high blood pressure, diabetes, and heart disease, all of which can hinder sexual arousal, performance, and pleasure.

Now that you understand the four key elements of great sex, here's our ten-step program to enhance sexual health and vitality.

The cooking couple's ten-step program for sexual health and vitality

Step 1:
Enhance your sexual vitality

While most species use sex purely for procreation, humans also use sex for recreation. Sex is a sport, and if you want to play the field, you've got to keep your equipment in shape.

Our Sex Rx:

Protein keeps you potent. Protein-rich foods contain tyrosine, an amino acid that the body uses to make the mood-elevating, sexually stimulating neurotransmitters dopamine and norepinephrine. Protein is also critical in making the hormones needed for sexual vitality as well as all body tissues, enzymes, hemoglobin, and antibodies.

While there is nothing wrong with the occasional T-bone steak (red meat is packed with zinc), try to keep your daily sources of protein lean: beans, fish, and poultry without the skin.

Go for ginkgo. Good old *Ginkgo biloba* has been around for over 200 million years and is the world's most ancient tree. The Chinese have been using the nuts and leaves for nearly 5,000 years to enhance sexual vitality, slow the aging process, and improve alertness and circulation. (People who are pregnant, nursing, or bleed easily shouldn't take ginkgo.)

Ginkgo works about an hour after it's taken to promote blood flow to the genitals for both men and women. The recommended

Lean and Mean

Red meat tends to be high in saturated fat and dietary cholesterol, both of which can raise blood cholesterol levels and clog the tiny arteries in your genitals and the blood vessels surrounding your heart. When you eat meat, stick to leaner cuts of beef—flank, sirloin, and tenderloin—and pork, such as tenderloin and Canadian bacon.

While the U.S. Department of Agriculture's (U.S.D.A.) Food Guide Pyramid says a serving of meat is two to three ounces of cooked, lean meat, we know that most people (especially Michael) would laugh at a serving size that small. Try to limit yourself to six-ounce portions, especially if you need to lose weight or lower your cholesterol.

You can make meat go further by thinking of it as a condiment and partnering it with vegetables in stews, stir-fries, casseroles, and kabobs.

Try replacing some of that animal protein with vegetable sources, including beans, soy, nuts, seeds, and whole grains. Not only will you avoid saturated fat and cholesterol, you'll add fiber as well as complex carbohydrates.

dose is 40 mg of 24 percent standardized extract three times a day.

When men with erection problems take ginkgo over several months, many experience improved blood flow, enabling them to regain their former level of sexual activity. According to a study published in the *Journal of Urology,* 50 percent of men with erectile dysfunction who took 60 mg of ginkgo extract daily for six months were able to have erections. Studies show gingko may also help reverse impotence for men on antidepressants (reversing impotence probably got them off antidepressants) and sexual dysfunction for women on antidepressants.

Ginkgo also improves the production of sperm and increases

Beans Boost your sex Life

The Romans may not have understood bean science, but they must have known something about the aphrodisiacal power of chickpeas, because they fed them to their stallions to keep them feisty.

Beans are rich in plant chemicals that keep blood vessels from becoming clogged. Just half a cup a day is enough. Here are some easy ways to incorporate beans into your diet:

•Toss a handful of chickpeas on your salad.

•Add beans to soups, stews, stir-fries, pasta dishes, and casseroles.

•Use textured vegetable protein (TVP, available in supermarkets and natural food stores), mashed beans, or ready-prepared vegetarian meat substitutes to replace all or some of the ground beef, pork, or turkey in recipes.

•Have a bowl of minestrone or black bean soup for lunch or dinner.

the production of neurotransmitters in the brain, which are needed for sexual arousal, response, and pleasure.

Dive in to clams and oysters. Not only are these tasty mollusks packed with vitamins and minerals that fuel great sex, they are a rich source of mucopolysaccharides, an aphrodisiac that increases sexual potency and libido.

Stop smoking. Okay, so it isn't dietary advice, but it is one of the best things you can do for your love life and your overall health.

Smoking decreases energy, sexual vitality, and libido by damaging blood vessels and limiting the amount of oxygen available to the body. Plus, smoking saps the body of nutrients like vitamins A, C, and E, which are needed for sexual vitality.

Heavy smoking also reduces sperm density and motility and can increase the risk of impotence by decreasing blood flow to the penis. And for you fans of oral sex, many women find the taste of semen from smokers unpleasant.

step 2:
increase libido

The male sex hormone testosterone is responsible for sex drive in both men and women and plays an influential role in orgasm and ejaculation. While testosterone levels drop as we age, the right diet helps keep levels high.

Stress can ruin your libido. Psychologically, stress makes you less interested in sex. Physiologically, stress diverts blood away from the genitals to tense muscles, making it difficult to become aroused and achieve an erection. Stress can also decrease fertility, cause testosterone levels to plummet, and lead to depression and anxiety, both of which diminish libido, sexual performance, and pleasure.

Satisfying sex, meditation, exercise, and consuming more nutrient-rich, unprocessed foods and less sugar and caffeine (which cause your body to crash after a high), can help you manage stress.

Our Sex Rx:

Hit the zinc zone. The prostate gland and sperm contain more zinc than any other part of the male anatomy. The body needs zinc to make testosterone and maintain vaginal lubrication. Plus, by increasing the production of T cells and improving white blood cell activity, zinc supports the immune system, helping you bounce back or avoid illness even when you are inundated by stress.

Foods high in zinc include: oysters, pumpkin and sunflower seeds, and lean beef.

Take ginseng. Ginseng was first used as an aphrodisiac by the Chinese and Koreans to enhance libido. Asian ginseng (also known as *Panax schinseng*) is best for improving sexual performance and energy.

Animal studies have shown that ginseng increases sexual activity, fertility, testosterone levels, and sperm production, and some human studies show it can help reverse impotence in men.

Ginseng is a tonic herb, which means it balances and strengthens many systems in the body (including the endocrine system, which produces sex hormones), improves energy and stamina, and helps us deal with stress.

For maximum effectiveness, ginseng needs to be taken over several months. The recommended dose is generally 100 to 200 mg a day. Look for a standardized ginseng formula that contains at least 5 to 7 percent ginsenosides (the active ingredient in ginseng). Stear clear of ginseng-fortified foods and beverages. They generally don't contain enough ginseng to make a difference. People with excessive bleeding and people on blood-thinning medications or diabetes drugs should not take ginseng without consulting their physician. Ginseng is also not recommended for people with heart irregularities and/or high blood pressure.

Vitamin C for sex. Vitamin C, the leading supplement in America, does more than ward off the common cold. It supports the adrenal glands, those little organs so vital in producing hormones that are key for sexual arousal and response, helps keep sperm swimming at an Olympic pace, and prevents male infertility.

Vitamin C also protects cells and sex organs from free radicals (destructive molecules produced in the body by a process called oxidation that can damage cells and lead to illnesses, including heart disease and cancer), boosts energy levels, increases the absorption of minerals such as iron, combats stress and infection, and reverses fatigue, a leading cause of libido lag.

Foods high in vitamin C include: citrus fruits (lemons, oranges, grapefruit, tangerines, and limes), cantaloupe, papaya, strawberries, peppers (chile and bell), broccoli, brussels sprouts, tomatoes, asparagus, cabbage, and leafy green vegetables.

Caffeine: use it, don't abuse it. Caffeine in moderation can actually increase libido. Coffee, which is a well-known aphrodisiac, can jump-start your day and your sex life.

Why do you think so many people meet for coffee on a first date? (More on this in Chapter 6, "Juicy Fruits." Yes, coffee is a fruit.)

According a study in *Archives of Internal Medicine,* coffee drinkers have sex more frequently and enjoy it more than non-coffee drinkers. A small study of older men found coffee drinking improved subjects' sex lives by increasing energy. Hot caffeinated beverages warm you up, wake you up, and are inherently social. Maybe the saying should be changed to "Coffee, tea, *and* me."

Like most good things, just a little is enough. Too much caffeine can stress the adrenal glands, which produce sex hormones; decrease testosterone levels; interfere with the menstrual cycle; and increase PMS. Try to limit yourself to about two cups of coffee, four cans of cola, or four cups of tea per day.

Drink alcohol in moderation. There's nothing like a glass of wine to relax you, loosen inhibitions, and put you in the mood for sex. (It increases the body's output of the libido-enhancing neurotransmitter dopamine.) Alcohol, in moderation, increases blood flow throughout the body and improves cholesterol levels.

However, too much alcohol can dull your senses, impair sexual response, and reduce testosterone production. So limit your intake to one or two drinks.

PENISES ARE GETTING SMALLER!

The average penis size reported in 1970 by the Kinsey Institute was 6.16 inches versus the 5.9 inches reported by the recent LifeStyle study. Is a secret government agency putting something in the water? Are the Russians stealing our mojo? John Holmes, come home! Calm down, boys. There is a simple explanation. While nurses measured the erect penises in the latest study, men measured their own size in the Kinsey study. What was Kinsey thinking? Any woman knows not to trust a man to tell the truth about the size of his penis.

STEP 3:
BUILDING A BIGGER, BETTER PENIS

According to a recent study conducted by LifeStyle condoms, the average erect penis is 5.9 inches long. The average flaccid penis is about 3 inches. Hard or soft, size depends on how much blood flows into your penis. More blood means larger, firmer erections that last longer.

Not satisfied with how you're hung? Many men aren't. Here are some safe, effective steps to make Mr. Happy happier.

Our Sex Rx:

Lose weight. The majority of the penis is anchored within abdominal fat, with only the tip protruding. If you are overweight, losing those excess pounds can give you up to an extra inch! According to Dr. J. François Eid, director of the Male Sexual Function Unit of New York Presbyterian Hospital, for every thirty-five pounds lost, penis length will increase by one inch.

While weight loss will not actually make your penis grow longer, losing weight will make more of the penis visible and us-

our top ten tactics to lower cholesterol

10. Eat less total fat (stay under 25 percent of calories per day).
9. Steer clear of saturated fats (stay under 10 percent of calories per day), trans fatty acids (hydrogenated oils), and cholesterol (stay under 300 mg per day).
8. Substitute more healthful unsaturated fats for bad saturated fats.
7. Eat garlic. Studies show it may help lower total cholesterol and raise good (HDL) cholesterol.
6. Exercise regularly. It can raise good (HDL) and may lower bad (LDL). Yes, sex counts as exercise. Has Mr. Happy done his push-ups today?
5. Don't smoke.
4. Eat more soy. Twenty-five grams of soy protein eaten a day as part of a diet low in saturated fat and cholesterol can lower bad cholesterol.
3. Control stress levels and your temper. Both can raise bad cholesterol levels.
2. Drink alcohol in moderation. It can help raise good cholesterol levels.
1. Eat more foods high in soluble fiber, like beans, apples, and whole grains, to help lower bad cholesterol. Aim for 20 to 35 grams of fiber a day.

able. Blood flow also benefits from weight loss, resulting in stronger and firmer erections.

Clobber cholesterol. High cholesterol nearly doubles your risk of erectile dysfunction (ED), a disease that, according to the American Medical Association, affects approximately 20 million Americans. A study in the *American Journal of Epidemiology* found that men with high cholesterol levels (over 240) have 1.83 times the risk of erectile dysfunction than men with lower levels. High cholesterol levels can also contribute to an enlarged prostate.

Eat arginine, the erection amino acid. L-arginine is an essential amino acid available in many foods, including meat, peanuts, chocolate, pumpkin seeds, almonds, and beef liver.

Studies show supplementing the diet with L-arginine can improve erections and sexual response in men. This amino acid is needed to make sperm and nitric oxide, a substance that makes erections possible. Viagra works by making more nitric oxide available when a man wants to have sex. In contrast, L-arginine increases the total amount of nitric oxide in the body. The suggested supplement dose is 2 grams twice a day.

Pump up your private parts. Women have long known that Kegel exercises (contracting the muscles surrounding the genitals) keep them sexually fit and toned. Men can also benefit from Kegels. According to one study of men with erection problems, 74 percent of them showed improvement and 43 percent were cured after doing Kegels for only four months!

STep 4:
FemaLe GenitaL and HormonaL Fitness

While female genital response to sexual stimuli is not as obvious as male response (the clitoris, like the penis, becomes engorged with blood), women need to have well-lubricated, aroused equipment to enjoy sex.

While testosterone fuels the sex drive, the balance of estrogen and progesterone allows a woman to respond to and enjoy sex when her libido calls. These two female hormones, when proportionate, keep the vagina thick and well lubricated, resulting in pleasurable intercourse, and stimulate the vulva, clitoris, and vaginal tissue to become excited during lovemaking. Plus, they influence a woman's mood and overall sense of wellness.

Many factors from stress to a poor diet can upset hormone levels. Research is starting to show that certain foods and herbs can actually help women strike a healthy hormonal balance so that sex remains exciting and enjoyable.

Our Sex Rx:

Soy for sex. Soy is the food darling of the new millennium. Studies show it can do everything from decrease cholesterol levels to prevent certain cancers.

But what's the scoop on soy when it comes to sex?

Soybeans are rich in phytoestrogens, plant chemicals that act like a weak form of estrogen. The plant estrogens found in soybeans can help decrease vaginal dryness and alleviate some of the symptoms of menopause that often dry up sexual desire.

Eat more EFA (essential fatty acids). The body uses essential fatty acids (EFA) to make female sex hormones, but the body can't manufacture them. They keep the vagina moist and soft and increase the storage of fat-soluble vitamins (A, D, E, and K), many of which we need to function sexually.

Women need two types of EFAs regularly: linoleic acid (omega-6) and linolenic acid (omega-3). Good sources of linoleic acid include soybeans; safflower, sunflower, and corn oils; wheat germ; and sesame seeds. Flaxseed, canola oil, pumpkin seeds, almonds and walnuts, and deep-sea fish such as tuna contain linolenic acid.

An easy way to get EFA is to take a tablespoon of flaxseed oil every day.

The joy of soy

Five ways to incorporate this wonder bean into your diet.
1. Substitute soy milk for cow's milk.
2. Try soy luncheon meats, hot dogs, burgers, and soy nut butter.
3. Snack on soy nuts or edame (fresh soybeans).
4. Add soy protein powder to your smoothies.
5. Learn to love tofu; its bland flavor lends itself to a wide variety of preparations. Add cubes of tofu to stir-fries and pasta dishes. Try it mashed in lasagna or other casserole dishes. Or mash it with herbs, spices, and a little soy sauce and sesame paste for a sandwich filling.

Pump up the pleasure with B₆. This B vitamin (aka pyridoxine) helps balance fluids and a number of hormones including estrogen and progesterone.

Like calcium, vitamin B_6 can help ease the symptoms of PMS. Increased levels of estrogen seem to increase the need for B_6, so if you are taking birth control pills or estrogen replacement therapy, consuming more B_6 may help alleviate symptoms such as vaginal dryness, loss of libido, fatigue, mood swings, and depression. However, do not consume more than 150 mg of B_6 per day in supplement form, as higher doses can cause nerve damage. There usually is no reason to get more than 25 mg per day.

Good sources of B_6 include lean red meat, liver, fish, chicken, egg yolk, wheat germ, bananas, prunes, avocados, soybeans, and walnuts.

Dong quai performs a balancing act. This herb, also known as angelica and female ginseng, is highly valued in traditional Chinese medicine as a female tonic. Like soy, dong quai contains phytoestrogens that can help regulate and balance estrogen levels. It is also prescribed to increase libido, treat menstrual disorders, and alleviate PMS.

Women who are pregnant or breast-feeding should avoid dong quai. It can also make some women more sensitive to the sun, so slather on the sunscreen if you decide to try it.

Dong quai is available in capsules, tinctures, and teas. For the correct dose, follow the package directions.

step 5:
attraction action: get a sexier, more attractive body

Let's face it, looking good is a magic elixir in one's love life.

Along with maintaining a healthy weight, there are a number of nutrients you can take and foods you can eat to beautify your body.

Our Sex Rx:

Start with A. Vitamin A (beta-carotene, which the body converts to vitamin A, and retinol, preformed vitamin A) promotes healthy, radiant hair and skin.

Vitamin A, like vitamin C, is also needed to make sex hormones. This fat-soluble vitamin keeps testicles healthy, enhances fertility in both men and women, and is used to make sperm. Plus, vitamin A promotes good eyesight, provides overall antioxidant protection, fights infection, and promotes healing.

Good sources of beta-carotene include orange fruits and orange and green vegetables such as carrots, yams, pumpkin, mangoes, apricots, brussels sprouts, broccoli, and kale. Liver, egg yolks, and dairy products contain healthy amounts of retinol.

The attractive acid. Want more attractive pearly whites to lure Mr. or Ms. Right (or Mr. or Ms. Right Now)? Then you need to add folic acid to your sexual supplement arsenal.

Taking 400 to 800 mg of folic acid a day or gargling with a 400 mg folic acid capsule dissolved in ½ cup water can reverse gingivitis and prevent bleeding gums and plaque.

Levels of folic acid tend to be low in women who are pregnant or on birth control pills or hormone replacement therapy.

Good food sources include leafy green vegetables, broccoli, folic acid-fortified breads and cereals, orange juice, and beans.

Eat blueberries and broccoli. Free radicals—unstable molecules generated by our metabolism and toxins in the environment that attack and damage the body and contribute to the aging process—can ruin your health and your looks.

Fruits and vegetables that are rich in antioxidants, such as blueberries, strawberries, oranges, plums, broccoli, spinach, and brussels sprouts, can prevent free radical damage and slow down the appearance of wrinkles, keeping you looking young.

Have more sex. Sex, particularly with a hearty orgasm, increases circulation throughout the body, giving you a healthy glow. Plus, lovemaking puts that mysterious je ne sais quoi smile on your face, and what can be more attractive and sexier than that?

step 6:
increasing sensitivity and sexual response

No two people have identical orgasms.

Fondling the G spot gets some women going, while clitoral stimulation turns on others. Some men enjoy just having their penis stroked, some crave having the entire genital area as well as the nipples stimulated.

There's no replacement for getting to know your body and

learning what works for your partner, but there are some nutrients that can help get the show on the road. To have better, more intense, and frequent orgasms, follow our diet advice.

Our Sex Rx:

Take niacin. Niacin helps to dilate blood vessels, contributing to a reaction called "the sexual flush," in which blood flows to the face, chest, and neck. The same blood vessel dilation also helps you achieve orgasm.

In addition, niacin enhances the sense of touch, making you more sensitive to physical stimulation.

Good natural sources of niacin include liver, fish, poultry, and peanuts.

Eat enough E. Vitamin E increases sperm production, helps ease PMS symptoms (especially breast tenderness), and increases fertility. E is essential in hormone production and balance. Vitamin E also helps keep your arteries clear, which means better blood flow, better erections, and better orgasms!

Increase dopamine. The dopamine/libido link was first discovered when patients with Parkinson's disease taking the medication L-dopa (which with the aid of magnesium and vitamin B_6 is converted into dopamine) noticed an interesting side effect. Their sex lives improved!

The neurotransmitter dopamine coordinates brain activities, including sex drive, emotions, and the ability to feel pleasure and pain. Kiss sexual arousal and orgasms good-bye without it.

You can increase dopamine levels in several ways:

1. Eating a protein-rich meal or snack will increase blood levels of tyrosine, an amino acid used by the body to make dopamine naturally. One to two grams daily of L-tyrosine broken up in three doses treats low sex drive. (Do not use without consulting your doctor if you have high blood pressure.)

Fava Knows Best

Fava beans are a rich natural source of L-dopa, which the brain converts into the neurotransmitter dopamine.

Hannibal Lecter liked his with a little Chianti, but you might try these ideas:

- Sauté fresh fava beans in a little olive oil and sprinkle with fresh or dried herbs.
- Add favas to pasta, rice dishes, soups, or stews.
- For a tasty spread, mash cooked fava beans with olive oil, garlic, and a little lemon juice.
- Look for roasted favas sold in gourmet food stores and ethnic groceries that carry Mediterranean foods.

2. Consume more folic acid, magnesium, and vitamin B_6, which the body needs to make dopamine.
3. Up your caffeine intake, which appears to increase the amount of dopamine in the brain by blocking adenosine receptors.
4. Reduce stress. Stress decreases levels of dopamine.
5. Eat fava beans.

Step 7:
Aromas for Amour

Sexual attraction starts in the nose. Yup, the nose.

People are attracted to each other by smell, a powerful, primitive sense that is processed in the limbic lobe, the emotional center of our brain. Since many of our first gratifying sensations are associated with food aromas, we are conditioned to expect pleasure when we smell foods that we love and associate with comfort and fond memories.

Humans can taste only sweet, sour, salty, bitter, and *umami,* a fifth type of taste recently classified and described as "savory, brothy, or meaty." So, in fact, what accounts for our ability to taste many complex flavors and combinations is actually our olfactory senses. Some 80 to 90 percent of what we refer to as taste is actually smell.

The nose knows.

While response to smell varies from person to person, research shows certain odors can put us in the mood for sex. In addition, the way our lover smells can turn us on or off. When your partner asks you to take a shower or hints that she likes a certain brand of aftershave, listen.

Humans, like other animals, secrete pheromones, odor-like substances that affect our behavior even though we don't consciously perceive them. Pheromones may be the magic element that causes love at first sight. (Or perhaps we should say love at first smell.) Scientists believe that pheromones are by-products of sexual hormones released from glands around the genitals and underarms that affect fertility, attract the opposite sex, and trigger sexual desire. Studies show that various pheromones may make people seem more attractive to the opposite sex and may keep sexual rivals away.

Two of the most studied human pheromones, the steroids androstenol and androsterone, resemble truffles, one of the most renowned aphrodisiacs, and musk, a scent commonly used in perfumes. Not surprisingly, the aroma of caviar, celery, and parsnips (all aphrodisiacs) contain androsterone and androstenol.

Other aphrodisiacs that smell like human pheromones include fresh shellfish, red wine, champagne, and pungent French cheeses.

Our Sex Rx:

Give her cucumbers and licorice. Certain smells can actually increase vaginal blood flow. The odor of Good & Plenty combined with cucumber increased vaginal blood flow by 13 percent.

Among women who reported becoming extremely aroused by masturbation, a combination of Good & Plenty and banana nut bread showed a 28 percent increase in vaginal blood flow (Get baking, boys!) according to research done by Alan R. Hirsch, M.D., director of the Smell and Taste Treatment and Research Foundation in Chicago.

Bake him a pumpkin pie. The smell of lavender and pumpkin pie increased penile blood flow by an average of 40 percent, followed closely by the smell of cinnamon buns. The smell of licorice and doughnuts increased penile blood flow by 31.5 percent. (Now you know why cops hang out at doughnut shops.)

Older men had a stronger response to vanilla, and men who were the most satisfied with their sex lives had a greater response to strawberries, according to the Smell and Taste Treatment and Research Foundation.

The sweet smell of success. Spike your breath with scents. According to Dr. Hirsch's research, 80 percent of women liked the smell of mint on a man's breath and 100 percent disliked the smell of alcohol. Of the men questioned, 42 percent (all of whom were single) preferred alcohol on a woman's breath, 30 percent liked mint, and 8 percent preferred chocolate.

From the Heart

Intimacy is good for the body, mind, and soul. One study of 10,000 individuals found that married men who felt loved by their wives experienced significantly less angina (chest pain). Another study found that wives who reported having a "deep emotional relationship" with their husbands had less coronary artery blockage than those who felt much less connected.

A Cooking Couple chocolate martini (page 315) with a mint chaser should do the trick for everyone!

step 8:
Enhance Intimacy

Intimacy is a state of being known by, and knowing, your lover. It is the glue that connects you to your mate and allows you to give and receive love and relate both sexually and emotionally. It enables you to feel comfortable together and more willing to share your sexual desires and needs.

Our Sex Rx:

Cook and eat together. Take out your calendar and mark two times in the coming week when you and your lover can share a meal. Prioritize and make time now.

"But . . . but . . . but what about my boss, my car, the dog, my cats, the peeling paint, the cracking wallpaper, the ball game, the work game, the lunch game, the get ahead game, the laundry, the lawn, my uncle John, and your mom? What will the neighbors say?"

Forget the excuses. Think of it this way: You're the doctor, and the problems are just going to have to sit in your waiting room until you get to them. Trust us, they won't leave. "Mr. Lawn, I'm sorry, the doctor is running a little late, have a seat and we'll get to you next weekend."

Set the problems aside and carve out some quality time or you'll have worse problems down the road.

The meal doesn't have to be fancy. (Simple and fun is fine.) The key is prioritizing intimate time.

Hint: Don't rule out breakfast and lunch for some fun. Why not call in sick and stay home for a romantic meal while the kids (if you have them) are in school?

cooking and Eating are Like Making Love

When you eat and cook, you use all of the same senses that you do when making love: smell, touch, taste, sight, and hearing. Tuning in to your senses in the kitchen and dining room warms them up for sex and increases your ability to listen to your body and your partner and experience pleasure.

Connect in the kitchen, then unite and ignite in the bedroom.

Feeling loved and nurtured builds intimacy and makes it much easier to open up sexually. That's one reason why food has always played a role in human mating rituals. When you cook for the person you desire, you communicate that you care as you nurture him or her at the most basic level of life.

Hint: Turn the heat up a notch and spice supper with an aphrodisiac or two. After dinner, head straight to the bedroom. Dishes? Forgetaboutit! In Cooking Couple land cleaning up means showering together.

Create rituals. Rituals make life meaningful by helping us pay attention to the moments that matter. The nightly dinner ritual, whether an elaborate meal or simple bowl of soup, restores and maintains a couple's or family's unity, security, and well-being. The dinner table is more than a place to simply feed.

We have created many rituals that force us to stop what we are doing and start enjoying each other's company. Because rituals are regular events, we have a built-in safety net to ensure that we focus on each other and spend quality time together. While sex is not always explicitly on the menu, the rituals create an aura of relaxation, pleasure, and connectiveness that usually leads to lovemaking. Plus, rituals keep sex and our relationship fun and interesting.

Some of our favorite rituals include:

- Opening a wonderful bottle of wine.
- Experimenting with aphrodisiacs. (That's how we discovered the Oyster Shooter on page 40.)
- Giving or receiving a massage.
- Buying special soap and taking a shower together.
- Dropping the kids off at Grandma's (one of our favorites).
- Planning, cooking, and eating a romantic meal.
- Listening to a new CD together or playing one of our favorite romantic CDs for each other.
- Conversing by candlelight.
- Playing strip poker.
- Modeling sexy lingerie. (Ellen walks, Michael stalks.)

Five Tips for Cultivating Compassion

1. Reflect on your own experience. Think about what makes you happy and causes suffering. How do you feel when your mate treats you with compassion, affection, and respect? Now, how can you do the same for your mate?
2. Put yourself in your mate's shoes. Recognize that like you, your mate wants to be happy and avoid suffering. This leads to a deeper level of understanding, connection, commitment, and a willingness to reach out.
3. Sit down together and make a list of ways each of you can be more loving. Put the list into action. Start by accepting your lover exactly as he or she is and take steps to boost his or her self-esteem.
4. Practice forgiveness. Remaining angry, resentful, and bitter requires tremendous effort and takes a toll on your physical and emotional health, so forgive and move on.
5. Joy and happiness are contagious.

Cultivate compassion. Compassion is the salve that can heal and transform your relationship and your life.

Compassion is the extension of the Golden Rule that we all learned as kids: "Do unto others as you would have others do unto you." True compassion is really a state of mind where you wish for good things to happen to your mate and for your mate to avoid suffering. When you identify directly with your mate's happiness, sorrow, and tribulations, your relationship deepens and sweetens as love and support come naturally from the heart and each partner puts the other first.

Like learning any new skill, developing compassion takes time. If you exercise compassion on a daily basis, at the end of the day you can go to bed at peace with your lover and yourself.

step 9:
Ditch PMS and UTIS

Urinary tract infections (UTIs) and premenstrual syndrome can kill romance. Most women don't want to make love when it hurts to urinate or when they are bloated, irritable, moody, or have a headache.

The good news is that you can decrease premenstrual symptoms with a few easy dietary changes. And while it is impossible to avoid UTIs altogether (most women get them occasionally), there are several things women can do to reduce their frequency.

Our Sex Rx:

Put the breaks on PMS with calcium and vegetables. Women who took 1,200 mg of calcium a day over three months decreased their PMS-related symptoms (depression, mood swings, irritability, headaches, ax murdering their partner) by half, according to a study published in the *American Journal of Obstetrics and Gynecology.*

Good sources of calcium include dairy products, broccoli,

canned sardines and canned salmon (which contains the bones), kale, soy foods, and calcium-fortified foods and beverages.

Women can fight PMS and menstrual cramps with a low-fat, completely plant-based diet. Researchers found that women who changed their diets saw results after only two menstrual cycles.

Try trading beef burgers for veggie burgers, switching from cow's to soy milk, and snacking on fruits and vegetables for a month or two.

Stay hydrated. Drinking plenty of water, at least eight 8-ounce glasses a day, can help prevent UTIs, or honeymoon cystitis, a painful bacterial infection that often becomes a problem when women go from having occasional sex to engaging in frequent lovemaking (which is bound to happen if you follow our advice on aphrodisiacs). Adequate fluids will also keep your skin looking good and your body functioning properly.

Drink cranberry and blueberry juice. Cranberry juice, cranberry supplements, and blueberry juice all help prevent and reduce the symptoms of UTIs by keeping bacteria from sticking to the urinary tract lining. A study published in the *Journal of the American Medical Association* found that women who drank 10 ounces of cranberry juice a day for one to two months significantly reduced the levels of bacteria that cause UTIs.

Step 10:
Prostate Preservers

When it comes to ejaculation, the prostate gland is a man's best friend, so take good care of him, boys.

During orgasm, the prostate gland secretes a fluid that mixes with and lubricates semen during ejaculation so those spermies can swim upstream like salmon in spawning season. If the gland becomes inflamed or enlarged, it can make sex and urination very painful as well as decrease the effectiveness of your sperm.

Each year thousands of men are diagnosed with prostate cancer, the treatment of which can cause sexual dysfunction. Many foods and pytochemicals have been shown to reduce the risk of prostate cancer.

Our Sex Rx:

Eat tomatoes and tomato products. Lycopene, the plant chemical that gives tomatoes, pink grapefruit, watermelon, and other fruits and vegetables their red color, helps prevent prostate cancer as well as cancers of the lung, colon, and breast.

Cooked tomato products, such as tomato sauce, tomato juice, and ketchup, are more effective cancer fighters than raw tomatoes. To boost lycopene's effectiveness, eat it with a little fat (a good excuse to order a pizza).

Soy solution. You can also keep your prostate humming by eating more soy foods such as roasted soy nuts, soy milk, and tofu. Cooking with garlic, rosemary, and turmeric or taking them as supplements can also help. While more research is needed, several studies suggest raisins may help preserve the prostate.

Saw palmetto can be a lifesaver. For men who are experiencing an enlargement of the prostate called benign prostatic hyperplasia (BPH), numerous studies have shown that taking the herb saw palmetto may reverse this potentially serious condition. Saw palmetto also seems to be more effective and have fewer side effects than drugs commonly prescribed for BPH. The recommended dosage is 320 mg of saw palmetto extract a day. Before you start taking any medicinal herbs or other supplements, consult your physician.

Putting it ALL Together!

Need more reasons to follow our plan?

When was the last time you went back for seconds?

You'll be less stressed and have more energy for sex.

You'll have greater sexual stamina.

You'll increase the amount of blood that flows to the brain, making you more alert for sex.

You'll also reduce your risk of heart disease, some cancers, and osteoporosis.

Whatever your food preferences, you'll find that many of the aphrodisiacs that we recommend easily fit into the Best Sex Diet.

The Quick Fix: The Cooking Couple's Get in Sexual Shape for the Weekend Food Plan

Whether it's a fourth date with Mr. Right and you want to be Ms. Ready or your fortieth anniversary and you want to remind her of that night at the drive-in when James Dean was on the screen and you were making the scene, our Get in Sexual Shape for the Weekend Food Plan will power-pack your sexual vault for Saturday night—or any night . . . all night long!

The foods and nutrients recommended here are designed to work quickly and synergistically to give you a swift libido lift. Although they are beneficial separately, by following our plan, you will maximize their effectiveness and your pleasure.

Monday: Go Nuts!

Saturday night is just a distant dot on the horizon. But it will be here sooner than you think (although not as fast as you would like). Today is the day you start to get ready for your amorous adventure. So instead of going nuts at work, grab some nuts and seeds and let them go to work on you.

Nuts and seeds are key fuel for great sex because they are rich in essential fatty acids, vitamins E and B_6, selenium, calcium, zinc, fiber, L-arginine, protein, and complex carbohydrates—all nutrients that boost sexual energy and vitality. Seeds and nuts help to make hormones and hormone-like substances called prostaglandins that are needed for sexual response.

If you or your partner have been on a very low-fat diet, you may be experiencing a libido lag due to a lack of essential fats. Nuts and seeds can quickly fix this problem.

Monday's Sex Rx for Men

Eat ¼ cup of pumpkin seeds today and every day for the rest of the week. Pumpkin seeds are rich in essential fats and one of nature's best sources of L-arginine, an amino acid that the body uses to make sperm and nitric oxide, essential to erections. Pumpkin seeds also nourish the prostate gland and are high in that all-important virility, fertility, and libido-boosting mineral, zinc.

Monday's Sex Rx for Women

Eat ¼ cup of nuts today and every day for the rest of the week. Three of our favorites are:
- Almonds. High in essential fats, fatigue-fighting iron, vitamin E, and some B vitamins. They have calcium, too, which will fight PMS.
- Brazil nuts. Your personal Latin lover, they are particularly high in the minerals selenium, which stimulates sexual energy, and manganese, which increases sex drive.
- Walnuts. Contain the key vitamins for sexual vitality A, C, E, and the Bs.

Tuesday: Herbal Enhancement Day

Tuesday is finger-lickin' good with herbs and spices that enhance your sexual vitality. Some of our culinary favorites are:
•Basil. Used in voodoo love ceremonies in Haiti.
•Cardamom. Take with milk and honey in the evening to fight impotence.
•Cloves. Considered an aphrodisiac in China since the third century B.C.
•Ginger. Works both internally and externally to increase desire and combat impotence.
•Nutmeg. Used as an aphrodisiac by the Hindus, Arabs, Greeks, and Romans.
•Saffron. We're just wild about saffron, which makes erogenous zones more sensitive.

For more ideas, see Chapter 8, "Enticing Herbs and Seductive Spices."

Tuesday's Sex Rx for Men and Women

Take either:
•Ginseng. Starting today, keep taking this sexual tonic and strengthening herb over several months to increase your overall health and sexual energy, or
•Ashwaganda. Used as an ingredient in sex tonics to treat impotence and a lagging libido, this herb can help increase blood circulation to the genitals. It also energizes and relaxes you, resulting in an improved overall sense of well-being. Start taking it now and take the recommended dose for two to three months. In addition, you should take
•Ginkgo. Studies show it increases blood circulation throughout the body, particularly to the brain and genitals. Take daily. Also pop an extra ginkgo tab about an hour before making love.

Tuesday's Sex Rx for Men Only

•Muira puama. This herb (aka potency wood) can increase sexual desire and make erections harder (hence its nickname). It has also been used traditionally to prevent baldness. Michael has always had plenty of hair, so we can't comment on its effectiveness in the coiffure arena.

Tuesday's Sex Rx for Women Only

•Dong quai. Also known as angelica, dong quai has been used in China for over 2,000 years. Along with balancing and supporting female hormones and alleviating PMS and menopausal complaints, dong quai can increase libido and sexual pleasure and intensify orgasms.

wednesday: c'ing is believing

Vitamin C nourishes the sexual organs and helps protect them from free radical damage, and it keeps sperm healthy. Plus, vitamin C will help you fight off colds and keep you energized for that big night out (or in).

Wednesday's Sex Rx for Men

Tone up with tomatoes. Eat a tomato or tomato products every day for the rest of the week. Not only are tomatoes rich in vitamin C, they are one of the best sources of the prostate-preserving phytochemical lycopene. So have sliced tomatoes on your salad or sandwich, take a V8 break, and drench that pasta with sauce. When Saturday night comes, you'll know why the French call tomatoes *pommes d'amour* (love apples).

Wednesday's Sex Rx for Women

Get fruity. Enjoy at least one citrus fruit or one glass of calcium-fortified orange juice—which will fulfill your daily C requirement—a day for the rest of the week. Actually, for the rest of your life. Oranges are a particularly good choice. They are also high in sexually enhancing folic acid and vitamin A.

Remember lemons. They help purify the body and are a great, low-calorie way to flavor salads and make water tastier.

Smooth Thursday

Two days until the big night. It's time to shake things up with our sexual smoothies. Whip up these delicious amatory elixirs to fuel your libido and turn on the afterburners.

Thursday's Sex Rx for Men

Drink one Testosterone Tornado. Stand back and watch out.

{ Testosterone Tornado }

2 tablespoons pumpkin seeds

1 cup milk or soy milk

1 scoop (2 tablespoons) protein powder

1 teaspoon instant espresso powder

1 ripe banana

2 ice cubes

Grind pumpkin seeds in a blender. Add remaining ingredients and blend until smooth.

Thursday's Sex Rx for Women

Drink one Estrogen Elixir. This potent beverage will whet your libido while it increases vaginal lubrication and secretions.

{ Estrogen Elixir }

1 cup soy milk

1 scoop (2 tablespoons) soy protein powder

1 tablespoon ground flaxseeds*

1 teaspoon cocoa

1 ripe banana

1 teaspoon blackstrap molasses (optional)

Dash vanilla extract

2 ice cubes

Combine all ingredients in a blender and blend until smooth.

Flaxseeds can be ground in a coffee bean grinder.

Free Fridays

Yes, you're free. Work and weekday responsibilities fade into the mist as Saturday starts to peek over the horizon.

Indulge yourself as you give your batteries a final charge and top off your sexual fuel tank. If you've got big plans for Saturday, stay home tonight, relax, and regroup with some self-indulgent care and high-octane fuel. Here are our Friday night menu suggestions to get you ready and randy for that big date.

Friday's Sex Rx for Men

The cocktail hour: A Bloody Mary (lycopene and vitamin C) spiked with plenty of Tabasco for an endorphin rush (see Chapter 4: "Chile Peppers") and a celery stick. (Celery contains female-attracting pheromones.)

{ Bloody Mary }

1½ ounces vodka

Dash of Worcestershire

Dash of lemon or lime juice

Tabasco or other hot sauce to taste

Celery salt and freshly ground black pepper to taste

Tomato juice

Celery stick (garnish)

Place several ice cubes in a tall glass. Add vodka, Worcestershire, lemon or lime juice, Tabasco or other hot sauce, celery salt, and pepper. Fill glass with tomato juice. Stir, taste, and adjust seasonings. Garnish with a celery stick.

The main course: Steak—rare and bloody—for the gladiator within, and a side of onions sautéed with garlic (both are famous aphrodisiacs) for your pre-weekend protein injection. Plus, you get healthy doses of zinc, iron, L-arginine, and a host of B vitamins.

Dessert: Dessert is for wimps. Pour yourself a large Scotch, pop a De Niro/Pacino double bill of testosterone into your VCR, sit back, crack some nuts, and watch how Bob and Al take care of business. Best pics: *Taxi Driver, Goodfellas,* any *Godfather* movie, *The Devil's Advocate,* and, of course, *Raging Bull.*

Friday's Sex Rx for Women

To start: Take a warm, relaxing bath by the light of a vanilla-scented candle while sipping a chocolate martini and fantasizing about your favorite men. (All at once, or one at a time. It's *your* fantasy, so let it go, girl!)

{ chocoLate Martini }

1 ounce vodka

1 ounce chocolate liqueur (such as Godiva)

Crushed ice

Cocoa

Combine vodka, chocolate liqueur, and ice in a cocktail shaker. Shake vigorously, pour into a martini glass, and sprinkle with cocoa. Yum.

The main course: Shrimp and tofu stir-fry with brown rice for high-quality protein, calcium, and complex carbohydrates to relax and energize you. Plus, the dose of soy can help balance your hormones.

Dessert: Rent a sexy or romantic movie while you nibble on Good & Plenty and cucumbers. Good chick flicks: *Woman on Top, Tom Jones, Like Water for Chocolate,* or anything with Hugh Grant, Sean Connery if you like 'em old and classy, or Ben Affleck if you like 'em wet behind the ears.

saturday Night speciaL

You're both well fueled to set sexual sparks flying. To keep the flames of love and lust stoked, here's our Precoital Saturday Night Special Menu for two.

To Start: Oysters on the half shell with champagne for light protein, plenty of zinc, and the right balance of expansive and contractive energy.

Next, assorted chocolates (why wait for dessert to get things rolling?) with your favorite licorice drink (for recipes, see Chapter 5, "Licorice and Its Kissing Cousins,") to increase levels of phenylthalamine (PEA), the love chemical.

The main course: Pistacho-Basil Salmon (see page 107) to provide you with the inspiration and energy for mattress-shattering sex.

{ general index }

{ R E C I P E   I N D E X }

About the Authors

ELLEN and MICHAEL ALBERTSON are the hosts of one of Boston's most popular weekly radio shows, *The Cooking Couple Show.* Ellen, a registered dietician and medical journalist, has written for such magazines as *Self* and *Natural Health.* Michael is a chef and comedian who has written for *Playboy* and *The Boston Herald.* They live in Boston.